INTERMITTENT FASTING FOR WOMEN OVER 50

The Complete Stress-Free Guide to Get Fit and Rejuvenate your body without giving up your favorite foods! Includes 21-Day Healthy Meal Plan & Workout

D1524174

TABLE OF CONTENTS

INTRODUCTION 4

CHAPTER 1: HOW TO DO INTERMITTENT FASTING? 7

CHAPTER 2: BENEFITS OF INTERMITTENT FASTING FOR WOMEN OVER 50 18

CHAPTER 3: HOW TO ACTIVATE ANTI-AGING PROCESS THROUGH INTERMITTENT FASTING 27

CHAPTER 4: VARIOUS INTERMITTENT FASTING PROGRAMS 37

CHAPTER 5: BEST WAYS TO LOSE WEIGHT AFTER 50 56

CHAPTER 6: DIETING AFTER 50 71

CHAPTER 7: NEGATIVE SIDE EFFECTS FROM FASTING AND HOW TO AVOID THEM 74

CHAPTER 8: HOW CAN YOU INCORPORATE FASTING INTO YOUR EVERYDAY ROUTINE? 87

CHAPTER 9: RECIPES 100

CHAPTER 10: 21-DAY MEAL PLAN 140

CONCLUSION 150

INTRODUCTION

Have you been trying to lose weight, but you've been having no luck? Are you older than 50? You're not alone if you're having trouble losing weight at this age. Women over 50 frequently see less success with weight loss. But this doesn't mean it can't be done; it just means you must understand why it's difficult and perhaps attempt a different strategy.

For women over 50, several factors can impede weight loss progress. Your body is now going through a drop in metabolic rate. This is driven by frequently decreased physical activity and a loss of lean muscle mass. Many older women find intermittent fasting a practical solution when trying to shed stubborn pounds.

Intermittent fasting has several positive health effects in addition to its possible function in weight loss.

Is Intermittent Fasting Beneficial For Women Over 50?

Women experience menopause in midlife, which alters their bodies in several ways. Losing weight is one of those things that gets tougher to achieve. So, is intermittent fasting safe for those over 50?

Weight increase in women during menopause is not unusual. This is due to the alteration in metabolism that occurs at this age. A decrease in progesterone and estrogen causes your metabolism to slow down.

In addition, insulin resistance may make it more difficult for you to metabolize sugars and carbohydrates. Fortunately, intermittent fasting for women makes it easier for your body to use belly fat for energy. Therefore, it may be easier to lose weight and keep it off.

What Is Intermittent Fasting?

Intermittent Fasting involves restricting meals to certain periods of the day or a certain period. You observe a period of fasting the remainder of the time. Once the fasting period is over, normal eating will resume. An illustration would be if you had an "eating window" where you could eat between 8:00 a.m. and 6:00 p.m. and then refrain from eating for 12 hours between 6:00 p.m. and 8:00 a.m. the following day.

There are a variety of intermittent fasting plans available for women over 50. Always consider your interests and lifestyle before deciding which approach would be the most effective for you.

CHAPTER 1: HOW TO DO INTERMITTENT FASTING?

Intermittent fasting has shown to be quite effective for a friend of mine. She loses weight by using intermittent fasting, and wow, has it ever worked. Her experience with fasting to reduce weight has persuaded me to give it a try myself. I'm not sure if I'll follow her intermittent fasting diet or not because there are so many different ways to achieve excellent weight loss outcomes with intermittent fasting. My friend Christine, who has had great success with her intermittent fasting diet, will eat every other day. She'll normally eat for twenty hours before fasting for the next twenty-four.

She began intermittent fasting for weight loss a few months ago and hasn't tried anything else. She had such positive outcomes that they motivated and encouraged her to keep going even when things were rough. This is great news because it's difficult for me to keep to diets, especially when they don't seem to work. When you fast intermittently, you see benefits rapidly, which is wonderful for motivation. Christine explained that the immediate results are the sole reason she could continue the diet because seeing the weight loss boosts your willpower. Because I've tried and stopped so many diets in the last few years, I desperately need one like this. Over the years, I've joined a number of organizations and associations, not to mention the money I've spent on them. I didn't start these diets and then quit them after a few days. I kept to every one of them for two weeks, and I decided the diet wasn't for me because I didn't lose any weight after that time. I gave up my favorite foods and modified my lifestyle, but I still didn't see any effects. I would have known something was working if I had seen any weight loss during that time, and it would have motivated me to keep with it. But that didn't happen, and I am still looking for the perfect diet. It will, hopefully, be intermittent fasting.

In recent years, IF has become a common health fad. According to devotees, it might lengthen their lifespans, improve metabolic health, and aid in weight loss.

Every approach can be helpful, but determining which one works best for you is a personal decision.

There are several approaches to manage this eating habit. However, before starting an intermittent fast or choosing how frequently to fast, you should see a healthcare professional.

Different methods of intermittent fasting exist.

1. The 16/8 method

The 16/8 approach involves reducing your daily eating window to 8 hours and fasting for around 16 hours each day.

Here, you're allowed to have two, three, or even four meals.

Fitness instructor Martin Berkhan pioneered this approach, also known as the Leangains program.

Following this fasting strategy is easy as not eating anything after supper and missing breakfast.

If you eat at 8 p.m., Fast for 16 hours, then eat again at midday the next day.

This strategy could be challenging for those who are hungry in the morning and want to have breakfast.

However, many people who skip breakfast eat this way naturally.

During the fast, you can consume water, coffee, and other low-calorie liquids to help you feel less hungry.

It's critical to focus on eating nutritious meals throughout your eating window. If you eat many processed foods or consume a lot of calories, this approach will not work.

The 16/8 technique entails 16-hour fasts every day. Eat just two, three, or more meals every 8 hours.

2. The 5:2 diet

According to the 5:2 diet, you should eat regularly five days a week and limit your caloric intake to 500–600 calories on two of those days.

This diet, commonly referred to as the Fast Diet, gained popularity thanks to British writer Michael Mosley.

Women should consume 500 calories on days when they fast, while men should consume 600 calories.

For instance, you may eat consistently every day excluding Mondays and Thursdays. For those two days, you have two moderate meals each with 250 calories for women and 300 calories for men.

The 5:2 diet helps assist in weight reduction.

The 5:2 diet, sometimes referred to as the Fast Diet, calls for eating 500–600 calories twice a week while eating normally on the other five days.

3. Eat Stop Eat

Eat Stop Eat involves a 24-hour fast once or twice per week.

Fitness guru Brad Pilon pioneered this approach, which has been extremely popular for a few years.

Liquids such as coffee, water, and other low-calorie drinks are tolerated during the fast, but solid meals are not.

You must keep to your usual diet throughout the eating periods if you're doing this to lose weight. In other words, you should consume as much as you would if you were not fasting.

A full 24-hour fast may be challenging for many people, which is a disadvantage of this approach.

Eat Stop Eat is a week-long intermittent fasting regimen that includes one or two 24-hour fasts.

4. Fasting on alternate days

Alternate-day fasting involves fasting everyday.

This technique is available in a variety of forms. During fasting days, some of them allow around 500 calories.

However, the few study that was conducted on the subject found that alternate-day fasting was no more effective than a standard calorie-restrictive diet for either weight loss or maintenance.

As a result, a complete fast every other day is not recommended for those just starting out.

This technique may cause you to go to bed hungry several times each week, which is unpleasant and unlikely to be sustainable in the long run.

Fasting every other day, either by not eating or eating only a few hundred calories, is known as alternate-day fasting.

5. The Warrior Diet

Ori Hofmekler, a fitness guru, introduced the Warrior Diet.

During the day, you consume modest portions of fresh fruits and vegetables, and at night, you eat one large meal.

You fast during the day and eat for four hours at night.

One of the earliest popular diets that involved a kind of intermittent fasting was the Warrior Diet.

The Warrior Diet recommends eating just modest portions of vegetables and fruits during the day and one large meal at night.

HOW MANY HOURS SHOULD A WOMAN DO INTERMITTENT FASTING?

The 16/8 model is the most common approach for intermittent fasting. That implies you'll fast for 16 hours and then eat for 8 hours.

The 16 hours are usually completed when you sleep, making it much easier.

This aids in hunger management and provides you with extra energy throughout the day. Experts offer the following advice on the process of intermittent fasting for women:

Skipping breakfast Intermittent fasting (IF), often known as time-restricted nutrition, entails skipping breakfast (TRF). IF is a food consumption pattern that alternates between fasting and eating at set intervals.

There are several ways to do it; one of the most popular is the 16/8 regimen, which involves fasting for 16 hours (usually overnight) followed by an 8-hour window to eat each day.

ALWAYS EAT AFTER 7 PM

Controlling hunger is most difficult before bed and first thing in the morning. You will have the most willpower to stick to the diet if you follow the Always Eat After 7 PM regimen because you will eat when you are most hungry.

INTERMITTENT FASTING FOR WEIGHT LOSS

The desire to lose weight is one of the most prevalent reasons people seek information about intermittent fasting for women. Always Eat After 7PM, a regimen created by Joel Marion, makes dieting simple and eliminates 90 percent of the reasons for resistance.

Based on unexpected research, always Eat After 7 PM debunks popular diet fallacies and provides an easy-to-follow diet that promotes fat-burning and allows you to indulge in your most intense food cravings: eating most of your calories at night.

HOW TO STAY MOTIVATED WITH INTERMITTENT FASTING

It's difficult to stay motivated when making a lifestyle change. However, one of the simplest ways to stick to it is to set up an intermittent fasting plan. One of the most effective strategies for staying on track is to plan meals and establish a schedule.

One of the easiest ways for me to do this is by eating between midday and 8 p.m. This enables me to have lunch, dinner, and a late-night snack. I don't get hungry until lunchtime after drinking a large glass of water with lemon for breakfast.

INTERMITTENT FASTING PLANS

Make sure to see your doctor before starting intermittent fasting. The actual practice is straightforward once you have his or her permission. You can choose a daily strategy, limiting your eating to one six- to eight-hour period each day. Try the 16/8 fasting method, which entails eating for eight hours and fasting for sixteen. According to one proponent of the daily routine, most people find it easy to maintain this pattern over time.

Another technique, the 5:2 approach, involves eating five times per week. You only consume one 500–600 calorie meal on the other two days.

Fasting for a longer period, such as 24 hours, 36 hours, 48 hours, or 72 hours, is not always healthy and can be very dangerous. If you go too long without eating, your body may respond by storing fat to compensate for the lack of food.

According to Mattson's research, the body adjusts to intermittent fasting in two to four weeks. You may feel hungry or irritable as your body adjusts to the new rhythm. He notes that research subjects which make it through the adjustment stage are more likely to stick to the diet because they feel better.

What can I eat while intermittent fasting?

You can drink water or zero-calorie liquids like black coffee or tea when you aren't eating.

And just because you're "eating normally" during your period doesn't mean you're "going normally." If you stuff your meal times with super-sized fried foods, high-calorie junk food, and desserts, you're not going to get healthy or lose weight.

On the other hand, Williams likes intermittent fasting because it allows her to eat — and enjoy — a wide variety of foods. "We want people to be conscious and enjoy eating wonderful, nutritious food," she explains. Eating with people and sharing the mealtime experience boosts happiness and promotes good health."

Like other nutrition experts, Williams believes the Mediterranean diet is a good model to follow, whether you try intermittent fasting or not. Choose complex, unprocessed carbohydrates like healthy fats, lean protein, whole grains, and leafy greens.

CHAPTER 2: BENEFITS OF INTERMITTENT FASTING FOR WOMEN OVER 50

Women over 50 can benefit from intermittent fasting to lose weight and reduce their risk of developing age-related illnesses.

Lower metabolism, achy knees, decreased muscle mass, and even sleep problems make it more difficult to lose weight after 50. Simultaneously, losing weight, especially dangerous belly fat, can significantly lower your risk of serious health problems, including diabetes, heart attacks, and cancer.

Of course, the chances of contracting various diseases rise when you get older. When it comes to weight loss and reducing the risk of developing age-related diseases, intermittent fasting for women over 50 can sometimes be a virtual fountain of youth.

How Does Intermittent Fasting Work?

You won't have to deprive yourself if you practice intermittent fasting, also known as IF. It also doesn't permit you to eat a lot of unhealthy food when you aren't fasting. Instead of eating meals and snacks during the day, you feed over a set period.

Most people adhere to an IF schedule that allows them to fast for 12 to 16 hours daily. They eat regular meals and snacks the majority of the time. Since most people sleep for around eight hours during their fasting hours, sticking to this eating window isn't as difficult as it sounds. You should also drink zero-calorie beverages like water, tea, and coffee. Fast Bars may also be eaten between meals to keep the fast going.

Build an eating routine that works for you for the best intermittent fasting results. Consider the following example:

• **12-hour fasts:** A 12-hour fast entails skipping breakfast and waiting until lunch to eat. You might eat an early supper and skip evening snacks if you want to eat your morning meal. A 12-12 fast is relatively easy to maintain for most older women.

- **16-hour fasts:** A 16-8 IF schedule will help you achieve faster results. Within 8 hours, most people prefer to eat two meals and a snack or two. For example, the eating window may be between noon and 8 p.m. and between 8 a.m. and 4 p.m.

- **5-2 routine:** You might be unable to stick to a restricted eating schedule daily. Another choice is to follow a 12- or 16-hour fast for five days and then relax for two days. For example, you might do intermittent fasting throughout the week and normally eat on the weekends.

- **Alternate-day fasts:** Eating very few calories on alternate days is another choice. For instance, you might restrict your calories to under 500 calories one day and then eat normally the next. It's worth noting that regular IF fasts never necessitate calorie restrictions that low.

If you stick to it, you'll get the best results from this diet. At the same time, you should take a break from this eating routine on special occasions. You should try different types of IF to see which one fits better for you.

Many people begin their IF journey with the 12-12 plan and then move to the 16-8 plan. After that, try to stick to your schedule as closely as possible.

What Makes Intermittent Fasting Work?

Some people claim that intermittent fasting has helped them lose weight simply because the small eating window forces them to eat fewer calories. For instance, instead of three meals and two snacks, they can only have two meals and one snack. They become more conscious of their foods and avoid refined carbohydrates, unhealthy fats, and empty calories.

Of course, you have the freedom to eat whatever healthy foods you choose. While some people use intermittent fasting to minimize their total calorie consumption, some use it in conjunction with a keto, vegan, or other diet.

The BEST Foods To Eat When You're Intermittent Fasting

Women's Intermittent Fasting Benefits Could Go Beyond Calorie Restrictions

Although some nutritionists believe that IF only works because it encourages people to eat less, others disagree. They assume that intermittent fasting produces better results with the same calories and other nutrients as traditional meal schedules. Studies have also proposed that fasting for several hours daily accomplishes more than just calorie restriction.

These are some of the metabolic changes that IF induces, which can help explain the synergistic effects:

• **Insulin:** Lower insulin levels during the fasting cycle will aid fat burning.

• **(HGH):** As insulin levels fall, HGH levels increase, promoting fat burning and muscle growth.

• **Noradrenaline:** When your stomach is empty, your nervous system sends this chemical to your cells to tell them they need to release fat for food.

Is Intermittent Fasting Healthy?

Is intermittent fasting a healthy way to eat? Remember that you can only fast for 12 to 16 hours at a time, not for days. You also have plenty of time to eat a delicious and nutritious meal. Of course, some older women may require regular eating due to metabolic disorders or medication instructions. In any case, you can talk to your doctor about your eating habits before making any adjustments.

Although it isn't fasting, some doctors claim that allowing easy-to-digest foods like whole fruit during the fasting window has health benefits. Modifications like these will also provide a much-needed break for your digestive and metabolic systems. For example, the famous weight-loss book "Fit for Life" recommended consuming only fruit after supper and before lunch.

In reality, according to the writers of this book, they had patients who only changed their eating habits by fasting for 12 to 16 hours per day. Despite not adhering to the diet's other guidelines or counting calories, they lost weight and improved their health. This technique may have succeeded precisely because dieters swapped fast food for whole foods. In either case, participants considered this dietary adjustment beneficial and simple to implement. Traditionalists won't call this fasting, but it's good to realize that you have choices if you can't go without food for more than a few hours.

Typical Intermittent Fasting Results

In the medical literature, Dr. Becky, a chiropractor and over-50 wellness coach, says it's difficult to find any drawbacks to IF. She demonstrated that the blood sugar and insulin levels would drop dangerously low during the fasting cycle. Your body will depend on stored fat for energy if insulin's hormonal fat-storing signal is absent.

The National Library of Medicine has also analyzed women's health-related sporadic fast outcomes. Studies on the use of fasting to minimize the risk of cancer, diabetes, and other metabolic disorders, as well as heart disease, are among the report's highlights.

Is Intermittent Fasting the Best Fat-Loss Tool for You?

In any case, IF seems to function primarily because it is relatively simple to follow. By reducing eating windows, they say it helps them naturally reduce calories and make healthier food choices. According to some research, IF tends to encourage fat loss while sparing lean muscle mass, making it a better option than simply reducing calories, carbs, or fat.

Of course, the majority of people combine IF with another weight-loss strategy. To lose weight, you might decide to eat 1,200 calories per day. It could be better to spread 1,200 calories over two meals and two snacks rather than three meals and three snacks. If you've had trouble losing weight because your diet didn't work or was too difficult to adhere to, you may want to try intermittent fasting.

Intermittent fasting (IF) is quickly becoming one of the most common methods for losing weight and getting lean and fit. Intermittent fasting for women and men is gradually gaining popularity as more people become aware of its benefits.

IF helps to increase vitality and endurance. The best part is that the outcomes keep you inspired. It is also said to help with cognitive function. Many people, however, remain suspicious of the method's usefulness because it is not suitable for all.

Longer fasting periods are not recommended for some women, even though shorter fasting periods are considered healthy for the majority of people.

CHAPTER 3: HOW TO ACTIVATE ANTI-AGING PROCESS THROUGH INTERMITTENT FASTING

Researchers discovered that restricting calories increased energy efficiency and reduced the risk of chronic diseases, including heart disease, diabetes, and cancer, while studying the effects of calorie restriction in overweight adults.

They discovered that calorie restriction reduced cellular damage and helped preserve stable DNA as they dug deeper. Since weakened and inflamed cells contribute to chronic disease, and aging begins when DNA wears down, these are two main factors in combating aging.

While calorie restriction has anti-aging benefits, most people cannot maintain a diet that reduces their caloric intake by 30-40% and sticks to it every day for a long period.

Intermittent fasting rapidly gained popularity as a viable alternative to calorie restriction. It provides the same life-extension advantages without the need for extreme dietary changes.

THE IMPACT OF INTERMITTENT FASTING ON YOUR BODY

Intermittent fasting causes the following changes, which function together to encourage a longer and healthier life:

Cellular repair: Cells expel further wastes that would otherwise kill the cells.

Gene expression: Genes that facilitate survival and disease prevention change.

Hormonal changes: Lower insulin levels prevent diabetes and can extend life expectancy.

Defends against inflammation: Intermittent fasting helps to reduce inflammation.

Protects against oxidative stress: Prevents cell damage caused by free radicals, which are reactive molecules.

Intermittent fasting also aids weight loss and the reduction of abdominal fat, which benefits your health and helps you avoid chronic diseases that can shorten your life.

DIFFERENT WAYS TO FOLLOW AN INTERMITTENT FAST

Many of our patients equate fasting with a difficult-to-follow deprivation schedule, but this is not the case with intermittent fasting. This method of fasting encompasses various eating plans that alternate between eating and fasting.

Here are a few intermittent fasting plans to get you started:

EAT-STOP-EAT

This scheme includes fasting for 24 hours once or twice a week.

16/8 METHOD (LEANGAINS PROTOCOL)

If you stick to this schedule, you'll miss breakfast, eat for 8 hours, and fast for 16 hours.

5:2 DIET

In this intermittent fast, you eat 500-600 calories on two non-consecutive days of the week. For the other five days, you eat a regular diet.

Fasting comes in a variety of forms and types. One intermittent fasting plan calls for eating days alternating with fasting days. Another variation on the 16/8 strategy is to eat for 12 hours and then fast for 12 hours.

BENEFITS OF THE PROLONG FASTING MIMICKING DIET

We suggest the ProLon Fasting Mimicking Diet at BioAge Health because we believe it is the best choice (FMD). The ProLon FMD, like all forms of intermittent fasts, is an ideal way to lose weight. And, like the others, it has anti-aging properties.

You go on a 5-day fast once every 1-6 months if you follow the ProLon FMD program. The difference is that you get the necessary nutrients you need during your fasting days, including limited energy calories, and the enjoyment of consuming ProLon FMD plant-based foods.

The prepackaged foods are clinically engineered to replicate the effects of intermittent fasting, so you can reap the benefits without feeling deprived. During your 5-day fast, the ProLon FMD program includes all the food, snacks, and dietary supplements you'll need.

THE PROPOSED HEALTH BENEFITS OF INTERMITTENT FASTING

Regarding weight loss, there are two theories as to why IF might be successful. The first is that "fasting periods cause a net calorie deficit, and as a result, you lose weight," says Rekha Kumar, MD, an endocrinologist, diabetes, and metabolism specialist at Weill Cornell Medicine and NewYork–Presbyterian in New York City. The other definition is more difficult to grasp: She believes that the so-called "plateau phenomenon" can be avoided by taking this approach.

You may recall the popular "Biggest Loser" report published in Obesity in August 2016. After six years, the researchers found that, after the initial impressive weight loss, the participants had recovered most of their weight and their metabolic rates had slowed, resulting in them burning much fewer calories than would have been anticipated.

While more research on the safety and efficacy of IF is required, one of its touted benefits is that it may prevent metabolic sputtering. "Most people who want to lose weight by diet and exercise end up falling off the wagon and gaining weight. Hormones that encourage weight gain, such as appetite hormones, are activated, and it's thought that intermittent fasting (IF) will help avoid this metabolic adaptation," says Dr. Kumar. Normal eating patterns in IF "trick" the body into losing weight until it reaches a plateau.

Diet, a Form of Intermittent Fasting, May Help You Lose Weight, Study Suggests

So, does it help you lose weight? Proponents of the proposal have agreed with a resounding yes based on anecdotal proof. "For people who can stick to IF, it works," Kumar says. However, proponents of the method argue that it is about much more than just getting a lean body. Lori Shemek, Ph.D., a Dallas diet and weight loss specialist and author of How to Fight FATflammation, tells clients that IF can improve insulin sensitivity (lowering the risk of type 2 diabetes), minimize inflammation, and "boost longevity by bettering the health of your mitochondria (cell powerhouses)," according to her.

Obese adults who followed IF for eight weeks lost an average of 12 pounds while lowering their total cholesterol, "bad" LDL cholesterol, and systolic blood pressure. The journal Nutrition and Healthy Aging published a study in June 2018 that showed that 12 weeks of IF didn't affect cholesterol levels, but it did lead to weight loss and lower systolic blood pressure. In October 2019, the journal Nutrients published a study of 11 IF trials in overweight or obese adults that lasted at least eight weeks. Nine of those researchers found that an IF program was just as successful in helping people lose weight and body fat as conventional dieting instead of limiting calories daily.

However, it's worth noting that researching human longevity is much more complex than studying weight loss. That's why, as in a report published in June 2018 in the journal Current Biology, much of the research that indicates IF promotes a longer life span has been done in animals, including fruit flies. Another study published in the New England Journal of Medicine in December 2019 indicated that the metabolic benefit of intermittent fasting is that it puts your body into a state of ketosis (the keto diet's metabolic state), where fat is burned instead of carbohydrates for energy. According to the researchers, the idea that ketones can activate the body's repair system, ultimately protecting against disease and aging, goes beyond the weight loss effects.

It's also crucial to keep the hopes in check. Since a lot of research is done on animals, it's more difficult to apply the findings to humans, who are more free-thinking and have to deal with the consequences of lifestyle problems like work stress, crazy schedules, emotional eating, and cravings, to name a few — that can make it difficult to stick to a diet. IF might be promising, but it's "actually no more successful than any other diet," according to a 2018 article on the Harvard Health Blog.

Who Shouldn't Try Intermittent Fasting

Not everyone can (or wants to) participate in IF. Women who are pregnant or attempting to become pregnant (extended fasting cycles can throw off the menstrual cycle), diabetics (blood sugar may drop too low in the absence of food), and anyone taking several drugs (food, or lack thereof, can affect absorption and dosage), according to Kumar. Also, if you have a history of eating disorders, adding times where you're "not allowed" to eat might set you up for a dangerous relapse.

It's important to be aware that IF has any side effects. Since low blood sugar can mess with your mood, you can be cranky — "hanger" is true — during fasting times. When you do eat, you must continue to eat a balanced diet. "One idea is that if you fasted for two days, it would be difficult to make up a calorie deficit, but in our culture, with access to calorie-dense foods, you could do it," Kumar says. Concentrate on nutrient-dense foods such as fruits, vegetables, lean meats, legumes, and whole grains (though some experts, like Dr. Shemek, also pair IF with low-carb or keto styles of eating). Expect low energy, bloating, and cravings for the first few weeks as the body changes, says Shemek.

CHAPTER 4: VARIOUS INTERMITTENT FASTING PROGRAMS

If you want to give it a shot, you have a few options for incorporating fasting into your daily routine.

Daily Intermittent Fasting

I follow Leangains' intermittent fasting approach, consisting of a 16–hour fast followed by an 8–hour feeding period. This method of intermittent daily fasting was popularized by Martin Berkhan of Leangains.com, where the name came from.

It doesn't matter when you start your eight-hour eating period. You can begin at 8 a.m. and finish at 4 p.m. Alternatively, you may begin at 2 p.m. and end at 10 p.m. You should do whatever suits you best. I've noticed that eating between 1 and 8 p.m. is the best time to eat. It's excellent because it allows me to spend time with friends and family at lunch and dinner. Breakfast is usually a solo meal, so skipping it isn't a big issue.

It's easy to get into eating on this schedule because intermittent fasting is done daily. You're probably eating at the same time every day and aren't even aware of it. It's the same with intermittent daily fasting; you simply learn not to eat at specific times.

One possible disadvantage of this strategy is that consuming the same number of calories throughout the week becomes more difficult because you normally skip a meal or two during the day. Simply put, training yourself to eat larger meals regularly is difficult. As a result, many people who try intermittent fasting lose weight. This might be beneficial or detrimental, depending on your goals.

I'm not a diet freak, even though I've been intermittent fasting for some time. I work on building excellent habits that guide my behavior 90% of the time to do anything I want the other 10%. What happens if I come over to watch the football game with you and we order pizza at 11 p.m.? I will eat it regardless of whether it's outside my feeding window.

Intermittent fasting done once a week or once a month is one of the best ways to begin intermittent fasting. Even if you don't fast to lose weight regularly, fasting has various health benefits.

For instance, Lunch on Monday is your last meal of the day. After that, you go without food until Tuesday lunchtime. This schedule allows you to eat every day of the week while still receiving the benefits of a 24-hour fast. It's also less likely that you'll lose weight because you are just cutting out two meals per week. This is an excellent way to gain or retain weight.

I've done 24-hour fasts before (most recently last month), and there are various ways to incorporate one into your schedule. The day after a large holiday feast is an excellent time to incorporate a 24-hour fast.

The ability to overcome the mental barrier of fasting is perhaps the most significant benefit of a 24-hour fast. If you've never fasted before, completing your first one will show you that going without food for a day isn't harmful to your health.

Alternate Day Intermittent Fasting (ADIF) (ADIF) entails longer fasting periods on different days of the week.

For example, you might have dinner on Monday night and then not eat again until Tuesday evening. You'd eat all day on Wednesday and resume the 24-hour fasting cycle after supper that evening. This allows you to go without food for long periods while still consuming at least one meal each day of the week.

This form of intermittent fasting appears to be widespread in research articles, but it isn't very popular in the real world, according to what I've seen. I've never tried alternate-day fasting and don't intend to do so shortly.

The advantage of alternate-day intermittent fasting over the Leangains method is that you can stay fasted for longer. In principle, this would increase the benefits of fasting.

However, I'd be concerned about not eating enough in practice. Teaching yourself to eat more consistently is, in my opinion, one of the most difficult components of intermittent fasting. You may have a feast for dinner, but it needs preparation, planning, and consumption. Most people who try intermittent fasting lose weight despite missing a few meals per week.

This isn't an issue if you are trying to lose weight. Sticking to the daily or weekly fasting regimens won't be too difficult, even if you're happy with your weight. If you are fasting 24 hours a day on multiple days per week. It will be difficult to eat enough on your feast days to compensate if you fast for 24 hours a day on numerous days per week.

So, it is better to try intermittent daily fasting or a single 24-hour fast once a month or a week.

16/8 INTERMITTENT FASTING: A BEGINNER'S GUIDE

Fasting has been practiced in many religions and cultures worldwide for thousands of years.

Fasting has taken on new forms recently, putting a modern spin on an ancient discipline.

16/8 intermittent fasting is a popular style of fasting. Proponents argue that losing weight and enhancing general health is a simple, practical, and long-term strategy.

This section discusses intermittent fasting (16/8), how it works, and whether it is good.

What Is Intermittent Fasting 16/8?

16/8 intermittent fasting involves limiting calorie-containing foods and liquids to a predetermined eight-hour window each day and abstaining from eating for the remaining sixteen hours.

This cycle can be done as often as you want, from once or twice a week to every day, depending on your preferences.

16/8 intermittent fasting has grown in favor in recent years, particularly among individuals wanting to lose weight and burn fat.

Unlike other diets, which typically have stringent limitations and regulations, 16/8 intermittent fasting is easy to follow and can produce genuine results with less effort.

It is often seen as less restrictive and more adaptable than many other diet regimens and may easily fit into almost any lifestyle.

In addition to promoting weight loss, 16/8 intermittent fasting is thought to improve blood sugar regulation, brain function, and longevity.

16/8 intermittent fasting entails eating just for eight hours of the day and fasting for the remaining sixteen hours. It may help with weight loss, blood sugar control, brain function, and longevity.

How to Begin 16/8 Intermittent fasting is simple, safe, and long-term.

To begin, choose an eight-hour window and limit your food consumption to that time.

Many people prefer to eat between 12 p.m. and 8 p.m. because it allows individuals to fast overnight and forgo breakfast while having a nutritious lunch, dinner, and a few snacks during the day.

Others prefer to eat between 9 a.m. and 11 a.m. between 9 a.m. and 5 p.m., leaving plenty of time for a nutritious breakfast around 9 a.m., a typical lunch around noon, and a light early dinner or snack around 4 p.m. before you begin your fast

You can, however, experiment to find the time range that works best for your schedule.

Furthermore, to optimize your diet's potential health benefits, limiting your eating periods to nutritious whole foods and beverages is critical.

Filling up on nutrient-dense foods can help fill out your diet and allow you to realize the benefits of this program.

Fruits: Apples, bananas, berries, oranges, peaches, pears, and so on.

Broccoli, cauliflower, cucumbers, leafy greens, tomatoes, and other vegetables

Quinoa, rice, oats, barley, buckwheat, and other whole grains

Healthy fats include olive oil, avocados, and coconut oil.

Protein sources include meat, chicken, fish, lentils, eggs, nuts, seeds, etc.

Even if you're fasting, drinking calorie-free beverages like water, unsweetened tea, and coffee will help limit your hunger while keeping you hydrated.

On the other hand, binging or overeating junk food may negate the benefits of 16/8 intermittent fasting and impair your health.

To begin 16/8 intermittent fasting, pick an eight-hour window and restrict your food intake to that window. Make sure to eat a nutritious, well-balanced meal during your eating period.

16/8 Intermittent Fasting Is a Common Diet 16/8 intermittent fasting is a popular diet because it is simple to follow, alter, and maintain over time.

It's also practical because it cuts down on the time and money you have to cook and prepare food each week.

16/8 intermittent fasting has been linked to a slew of health benefits, including Increased weight loss: Not only can limiting your consumption to a few hours per day help you consume fewer calories throughout the day, but studies also show that fasting can stimulate metabolism and help you lose weight.

Fasting insulin levels can be reduced by up to 31% and blood sugar levels by 6% with intermittent fasting.

While human data is sparse, certain animal studies have discovered that intermittent fasting may increase longevity.

16/8 intermittent fasting is simple, adaptable, and convenient. Animal and human research suggest that it may help with weight loss, blood sugar levels, brain function, and longevity.

While 16/8 intermittent fasting offers many health benefits, it also has certain negatives and may not suit everyone.

Limiting your intake to only eight hours per day may encourage some to eat more than usual during meal periods to compensate for fasting hours.

This can result in weight gain, digestive issues, and the formation of poor eating habits.

16/8 intermittent fasting may also create short-term negative side effects, such as hunger, weakness, and exhaustion when you first begin; however, these usually fade once you get into a rhythm.

Furthermore, some evidence suggests that intermittent fasting affects men and women differently, with animal studies indicating that it may interfere with female fertility and reproduction.

However, more human research is needed to assess the impact of intermittent fasting on reproductive health.

In any event, begin gently and consider discontinuing or consulting your doctor if you have any worries or encounter negative symptoms.

Daily food restriction might result in weakness, hunger, increased food consumption, and weight gain. In animal experiments, intermittent fasting has been shown to have different effects on males and women and may even interfere with reproduction.

Is Intermittent Fasting (16/8) a Good Fit for You?

16/8 intermittent fasting, when combined with a nutritious diet and a healthy lifestyle, can be a sustainable, safe, and simple technique for improving your health.

However, it should not be considered a replacement for a well-balanced, well-rounded diet rich in whole foods. Furthermore, you can still be healthy even if intermittent fasting does not work for you.

Although 16/8 intermittent fasting is usually considered safe for most healthy adults, you should see your doctor before doing it, particularly if you have any underlying health conditions.

This is very important if you have diabetes, low blood pressure, or a history of disordered eating.

Contraceptive, pregnant, or nursing women should avoid intermittent fasting.

Consult your doctor if you have negative side effects during fasting. 16/8 intermittent fasting entails eating for eight hours and fasting for the remaining sixteen.

It may help with weight loss, blood sugar control, brain function, and longevity.

Consume a nutritious diet and drink calorie-free liquids such as water, unsweetened teas, and coffee during your eating period.

Before attempting intermittent fasting, speak with your doctor, especially if you have any underlying health issues.

6 POPULAR INTERMITTENT FASTING METHODS

Intermittent fasting has recently become a health craze. Its devotees claim it can help them lose weight, improve metabolic health, and possibly even live longer.

Every strategy can be helpful, but determining which one works best for you is a personal decision.

This eating pattern can be approached in a variety of ways. However, you should see a healthcare expert before beginning an intermittent fast or deciding how often to fast.

Intermittent fasting can be done in six different ways.

1. The 16/8 method

The 16/8 approach entails fasting for roughly 16 hours each day and limiting your daily eating window to approximately 8 hours.

Mealtimes are flexible and allow for multiple meals.

Fitness instructor Martin Berkhan pioneered this strategy, also known as the Leangains regimen.

It's as easy as not eating anything after dinner and skipping breakfast to follow this fasting method.

If you eat your final meal at 8 p.m., you'll have fasted for 16 hours by midday the next day.

This strategy may be difficult for persons hungry in the morning and who like to have breakfast. Many breakfast-skippers, on the other hand, eat in this manner instinctively.

During the fast, you can drink water, coffee, and other low-calorie liquids to help you feel less hungry.

It's critical to focus on eating healthy foods within your eating window. If you eat many processed foods or consume a lot of calories, this strategy will not work.

The 16/8 technique entails 16-hour fasts every day. You'll eat two, three, or more meals in 8 hours daily.

2. The 5:2 diet

The 5:2 diet consists of eating what you normally eat five days a week and lowering your calorie intake to 500–600 calories two days a week.

Michael Mosley, a British journalist, popularized this regimen, also known as the Fast Diet.

On fasting days, ladies should consume 500 calories, and males should consume 600 calories.

You might, for example, normally eat every day except Mondays and Thursdays. Every day, you consume two small meals of 250 calories for women and 300 calories for males.

The 5:2 diet is useful in assisting weight loss.

The 5:2 diet, often known as the Fast Diet, consists of eating 500–600 calories for two days of the week and regularly eating for the remaining five days.

3. Eat Stop Eat

Sometimes a 24-hour fast is required.

Fitness instructor Brad Pilon introduced this strategy, which has been fairly popular for a few years.

Fasting from one dinner to the next is equivalent to a full 24-hour fast.

Suppose you complete dinner at 7 p.m., for example. Monday, don't eat until 7 p.m. for supper. You've just finished a full 24-hour fast on Tuesday. The outcome is the same whether you fast from breakfast to lunch or lunch to lunch.

Liquids such as water, coffee, and other low-calorie beverages are tolerated during the fast, but solid foods are not.

You must keep to your regular diet during the eating periods if you're doing this to lose weight. In other words, you should eat as much as you would if you weren't fasting.

A full 24-hour fast may be challenging for many people, which is a possible disadvantage of this strategy. You don't have to go all in straight away, though. Starting with 14–16 hours and working your way up is fine.

Eat Stop Eat is a week-long intermittent fasting program that includes one or two 24-hour fasts.

4. Alternate-day fasting

Alternate-day fasting is intermittent fasting in which you fast every other day.

This approach is available in a variety of forms. During fasting days, some of them allow roughly 500 calories.

However, a small study indicated that alternate-day fasting was no more successful than a traditional calorie-restrictive diet for weight loss or maintenance.

A complete fast every other day may seem excessive, so it is not recommended for beginners.

This strategy may cause you to go to bed hungry several times each week, which is unpleasant and unlikely to be sustainable in the long run.

Fasting every other day, either by not eating or eating only a few hundred calories, is known as alternate-day fasting.

5. The Warrior Diet

The Warrior Diet Ori Hofmekler, a fitness specialist, introduced the Warrior Diet.

During the day, you consume little amounts of raw fruits and vegetables, and at night, you eat one large meal.

You fast during the day and eat inside a 4-hour eating window at night.

One of the earliest popular diets to involve a sort of intermittent fasting was the Warrior Diet.

The food options on this diet are quite similar to those on the paleo diet, consisting largely of complete, unprocessed foods.

The Warrior Diet recommends eating only small amounts of vegetables and fruits during the day and one large meal at night.

6. Spontaneous meal skipping

You don't have to follow a structured intermittent fasting schedule to gain some of the benefits of intermittent fasting. Another option is to skip meals when you aren't hungry or too busy to make and eat.

On the other hand, some people eat every few hours to avoid starvation or losing muscle. Others' bodies are built to withstand extended periods of starvation and occasionally go without one or two meals. Only you genuinely understand yourself.

So, if you're not hungry one day, skip breakfast and eat a nutritious lunch and dinner instead. You might be able to do a short fast if you're traveling and can't find anything you want to eat.

A spontaneous intermittent fast is when you skip one or two meals when you feel like it.

During the non-fasting periods, be sure you consume nutritious, balanced meals.

CHAPTER 5: BEST WAYS TO LOSE WEIGHT AFTER 50

Living a healthy lifestyle or shedding excess body fat can be difficult for some people as they age. Weight gain after age 50 can be caused by unhealthy habits, a primarily sedentary lifestyle, poor food choices, and metabolic changes.

By making a few easy changes, you may lose weight at any age, irrespective of your physical abilities or medical conditions.

Here are the top 20 weight-loss strategies for those over 50.

1. Get into the habit of enjoying strength exercise.

Strength training is particularly crucial for older folks, even if cardio gets a lot of attention in weight loss.

Sarcopenia is a condition in which your muscle mass decreases as you age. Around 50, muscle mass loss starts, which can reduce your metabolism and cause weight gain.

After 50, your muscle mass reduces by roughly 12% annually, while your muscular strength starts to decline at a rate of 1.5–5% per year.

As a result, muscle-building exercises in your workout program are critical for preventing age-related muscle loss and maintaining a healthy body weight.

Bodyweight workouts and weightlifting, for example, can develop muscular strength and growth while also increasing muscle function.

Strength training can also help you shed weight by reducing body fat and increasing your metabolism, which can help people burn more calories throughout the day.

2. Form a group

It can be difficult to independently establish a healthy eating habit or exercise routine. Keeping to your plan and accomplishing your wellness objectives may be easier if you team up with a friend, coworker, or family member.

According to studies, people participating in weight-reduction programs with friends are likelier to keep their weight loss over time.

Working out with friends can also help you stay committed to your fitness regimen and make it more fun.

3. Move more and sit less.

To lose fat in the body, you must burn more calories than you consume. That is why being more energetic throughout the day is important when attempting to reduce weight.

For example, sitting at your desk for long periods may sabotage your weight loss attempts. To combat this, standing up from your desk and enjoying a five-minute stroll every hour will help you become much more active at work.

According to studies, using a pedometer or Fitbit to count your steps can help you lose weight by improving your activity and calorie burning.

Begin with a reasonable step target depending on your current activity levels while using a pedometer or Fitbit. Then, based on your overall health, progressively increase to 7,000–10,000 steps per day or more.

4. Increase your protein consumption.

It's vital to have enough high-quality protein in your diet not just for weight loss but also to prevent or reverse age-related muscle loss

After the age of 20, your resting metabolic rate (RMR), or the number of calories you burn at rest, declines by 1–2% per decade. This is linked to muscle loss as people get older.

On the other hand, a protein-rich diet can help avoid or even prevent muscle loss. Various studies have also proved dietary supplementation protein helps you lose weight and keep it off in the long run.

Furthermore, research reveals that older persons require more protein than younger adults, emphasizing the importance of including protein-rich foods in your snacks and meals.

5. Consult a dietician

Finding an eating routine that supports weight loss while nourishing your body might be tough. A licensed dietician can help determine the most effective strategy to lose excess body fat while adhering to a strict diet. A nutritionist can also help you lose weight by providing support and guidance.

According to research, working with a nutritionist to reduce weight can produce much better outcomes than trying it alone. It may also help you maintain your weight reduction over time.

6. Prepare more meals at home

Various studies have shown that persons who eat more meals at home have a healthier diet and are less overweight than those who do not. When you prepare meals at home, you have complete control over what goes into and stays out of your recipes. It also lets you try out new, nutritious ingredients that have piqued your attention.

Start with preparing one or two food at home per week if you eat out almost all the time, and start increasing this number until you're preparing a meal more than you eat.

7. Consume more fruits and vegetables

Vegetables and fruits are high in nutrients essential for good health, and including them in your diet is a simple, scientifically proven strategy to lose weight.

A study of ten research indicated that increasing daily vegetable servings were linked to a decreased 0.14-inch (0.36-cm) waist circumference in women.

Another study found that eating veggies and fruits lowered body weight, waist circumference, and body fat in 26,340 women and men aged 35–65.

8. Engage the services of a personal trainer.

Engaging with a personal trainer can be extremely beneficial for individuals new to working out since they can show you how to exercise properly to lose weight and avoid injury.

Personal trainers can also encourage you to exercise more by holding you responsible. They might even change your mind about working out.

10-week research of 129 participants found that 1 hour of one-on-one personal training each week enhanced exercise interest and physical activity levels.

9. Reduce your reliance on convenience foods.

Consuming convenience meals like fast food, candies, and junk foods regularly have been linked to weight gain and may sabotage your weight loss attempts.

Convenience foods are rich in calories and poor in critical elements such as fiber, protein, vitamins, and minerals. Fast food and other processed foods are sometimes referred to as "empty calories."

Reducing convenience foods and substituting them with nutrient-dense whole foods in healthful meals and snacks is a good strategy to reduce weight.

10. Find something you enjoy doing.

Finding a fitness plan you can stick to for the long haul might be challenging. This is why it's critical to participate in things you enjoy.

Sign up for a group sport like running or soccer, for instance, if you enjoy group activities. This will allow you to exercise with others regularly.

If you like solo activities, go for a solo bike ride, a solo stroll, a solo hike, or a solo swim.

11. Have your health tested by a professional.

Suppose you're having trouble losing weight despite being active and eating a nutritious diet. In that case, you should rule out illnesses that make it harder to lose weight, such as hypothyroidism and polycystic ovary syndrome (PCOS).

This is especially true if you have family members who suffer from these ailments. Tell your doctor about your symptoms so he or she can choose the appropriate testing procedure to rule out any medical disorders causing your weight loss problems.

12. Consume a diet rich in whole foods.

Following a diet rich in whole foods is the simplest method to guarantee that your body receives the nutrients required to thrive.

Whole foods, such as vegetables, fruits, nuts, seeds, chicken, legumes, fish, and grains, are high in fiber, protein, and fats, which are important for maintaining a healthy body weight.

In numerous studies, whole-food-based diets, both plant-based and those containing animal products, have been linked to weight loss.

13. Consume fewer calories at night.

Many studies show that eating fewer calories at night can help you stay healthy and shed fat.

Over six years, those who consumed more calories at supper were more than twice as likely to become obese than those who consumed more calories earlier in the day, according to a study of 1,245 adults.

Furthermore, those who consumed more calories at supper were more likely to develop metabolic syndrome, a combination of disorders that include elevated blood sugar and extra abdominal fat. Heart disease, diabetes, and stroke are all increased by metabolic syndrome.

Breakfast and lunch should contain most of your calories, with a lighter dinner being a viable option for weight loss.

14. Pay attention to your body composition.

Though your body weight is an excellent measure of health, your body composition, the percentages of fat and fat-free mass in your body — is also significant.

Muscle mass, particularly in older persons, is a significant indicator of general health. Your objective should be to gain more muscle while decreasing fat.

There are several methods for calculating your amount of body fat. Measuring your waist, calves, chest, biceps, and thighs, on the other hand, can assist you in figuring out if you're losing fat and building muscle.

15. Drink plenty of water in a healthy manner.

Drinks contain added sugars and calories, such as sweetened coffee beverages, juices, soda, sports drinks, and pre-made smoothies.

Sweetened beverages, particularly those fortified with high-fructose corn syrup, have been related to weight gain and obesity, diabetes, heart disease, and fatty liver disease.

Substituting healthy liquids like water and herbal tea for sugary beverages will help weight loss and lower your risk of acquiring the chronic illnesses listed above.

16. Select the appropriate supplements

If you're tired and unmotivated, the correct vitamins can help you get the energy you need to achieve your objectives.

Your capacity to absorb some nutrients decreases as you age, raising your risk of deficiency. According to the study, adults over 50, for example, frequently lack folate and vitamin B12, two elements required for energy synthesis.

B vitamin deficiencies, such as B12 deficiency, can affect your mood, create fatigue, and prevent weight loss.

As a result, adults over 50 should take a high-quality B-complex vitamin to help reduce the risk of insufficiency.

17. Limit added sugars

For losing weight at any age, avoiding foods high in added sugar, such as sweetened beverages, sweets, cakes, cookies, ice cream, sweetened yogurts, and sugary cereals, is crucial. Considering sugar is added to so many meals, even things you would still not expect, like tomato sauce, salad dressing, and bread, reading the ingredient labels is the best method to determine if something has added sugar.

Look for "added sugars" on the nutrition facts label or for typical sweeteners like cane sugar, high-fructose corn syrup, and agave in the ingredient list.

18. Improve the quality of your sleep

Your weight loss efforts may be harmed if you don't get enough good sleep. Sleep deprivation has been connected to an increased risk of obesity and has been shown to sabotage weight control efforts in numerous research.

A two-year study of 245 women discovered that those who slept 7 hours or more per night were 33% less likely to gain weight than others who slept less than 7 hours each night. Weight loss effectiveness was also linked to better sleep quality.

Reduce the light in your bedroom and avoid using your phone or watching TV before bed to get the required 7–9 hours of sleep every night and enhance your sleep habits.

19. Experiment with intermittent fasting.

IF is an eating pattern in which you can only eat for a certain time. The 16/8 approach, in which you eat for 8 hours and then fast for 16, is the most common type of intermittent fasting.

Intermittent fasting has been demonstrated to help people lose weight in numerous studies.

Furthermore, some test-tube and animal research suggests that intermittent fasting may help older humans by extending life, reducing cell decline, and preventing age-related alterations to mitochondria, your cells' energy-producing organelles.

20. Be more aware

Mindful eating is a simple method to enhance your connection with food while also helping you lose weight.

Mindful eating entails paying closer attention to what you eat and how you eat. It helps you understand your hunger and fullness cues and how food affects your mood and overall well-being.

Many studies have found that mindful eating helps people lose weight and improve their eating habits.

There are no hard and fast rules for mindful eating, but eating slowly, paying enough attention to the flavor and aroma of each bite, and taking note of how you feel throughout meals are simple methods to start.

Last but not least though it may appear that weight loss becomes more difficult as you get older, several evidence-based treatments can help you accomplish and maintain healthy body weight after 50.

Cutting added sugars from your diet, including strength training in your exercises, eating more protein, preparing meals at home, and eating a whole-food-based diet are just a few of the ways you may enhance your general health and shed excess body fat.

Try the suggestions above, and you'll find that losing weight after 50 is a delight.

CHAPTER 6: DIETING AFTER 50

At any age, maintaining a healthy weight is a worthy objective. It might be more difficult as you grow older.

You might not burn as many calories as you were younger, but you can still lose weight.

The weight-loss golden guidelines still apply:

- You should burn more calories than you consume.

- Keep meat and poultry lean by eating more vegetables, fruits, whole grains, fish, legumes, and low-fat or fat-free dairy.

- Sugars and meals with little or no nutritional value should be avoided.

- Fad diets aren't worth it since the outcomes aren't long-lasting.

If you're over 50 and want to reduce weight, there are a few extra things you should do.

1. Maintain your strength

As you become older, you lose muscle mass. Strength training can help to compensate for this. In yoga and

Pilates, you can utilize weight machines at the gym, lesser weights held in your hands, or your body weight for resistance. According to Joanna Li, RD, a nutritionist at Foodtrainers in New York, maintaining muscle mass is crucial to burning more calories.

"If you continue to eat the same manner you did when you were 25, you will undoubtedly acquire weight." — RD Joanna Li

2. Increase your protein intake

Because you're in danger of losing muscle mass, incorporate one gram of protein every kilogram (2.2 pounds) of body weight into your diet. "Protein also helps with weight reduction attempts since it keeps you full for longer," Li explains. Wild salmon, whole eggs, organic whey protein powder, and grass-fed beef are among the foods she suggests.

3. Drink plenty of water.

According to Li, you may not recognize when you're thirsty as quickly as you become older. She recommends drinking 64 ounces of water every day. You may drink or obtain a portion of it from foods like cucumbers and tomatoes, naturally high in water. Check your pee if you're not sure you're getting enough water: it should be light yellow.

4. Get a Leg Up on Your Metabolism

Eat smaller meals and snacks more often, and don't spend more than 3 hours without eating. "Because your metabolism is already sluggish, starving yourself slows it down," Li explains. You might not need as many calories as you did younger. Consult your doctor or a trained nutritionist for further information. "If you eat the same way you did when you were 25, you will acquire weight," Li warns.

CHAPTER 7: NEGATIVE SIDE EFFECTS FROM FASTING AND HOW TO AVOID THEM

It's still uncertain if intermittent fasting (and how it affects the body on a cellular level, for example) or calorie restriction is the root cause of the alleged benefits. So far, it's a case of trial and error to see if an IF eating style is right for you and your body.

On the other hand, IF has several potential negative side effects.

As previously stated, the benefits of intermittent fasting are still being studied, but there are some positive results. However, there is plenty of anecdotal evidence that IF has some potentially harmful side effects, and you should discuss them with your doctor before embarking on an IF eating plan.

Here are ten red flags to be aware of. If you experience any of these side effects, you should immediately pause IF and consult with your doctor or a nutritionist before continuing.

1. Feeling hangry

We're not sure if "hangriness" is a real term, but it is undoubtedly a real sensation. This is the grumpiness, irritability, or general irritability that comes from not eating while your body indicates that you are hungry.

As previously stated by WH, training the body to go 16 hours without food requires practice, and some people's bodies can never be satisfied with eating within such a narrow window.

In principle, you shouldn't be hungry first thing in the morning if you eat enough protein later in the day or at night. If you are, it's a sign that you need to make some dietary changes during your calorie intake cycle to stop being a total jerk—or it's a sign that fasting isn't working for you. Not eating for long periods might not be suitable for certain people (e.g., those who work out a lot), which is worth considering. Don't try to push it.

2. Fatigue or brain fog

Have you ever woken up in the middle of the morning, yawning uncontrollably, only to realize you'd forgotten to eat breakfast? As most people do IF by skipping breakfast, noticing that you're always tired—or making mistakes because of brain fog—is a sign that you're not consuming the right foods during non-fasting hours or that fasting isn't working for you.

"Pay attention to what you're putting into your body," Koens advises. "On IF, you can eat whatever you want, but you should still fuel it with nutritious foods that make you feel safe and strong." Listen to your body if you simply feel *much* healthier eating breakfast most days.

3. Food obsessions

According to Koens, a restricted diet may affect your relationship with food. While some people enjoy the strictness of IF, others can obsess about what they should eat and how many calories they consume.

Spending too much time worrying about the quality or quantity of your food daily can lead to orthorexia, a form of an eating disorder. According to the National Eating

Disorders Association, orthorexia is a condition in which you place such a high value on "right" or "healthy" eating that it negatively impacts your overall health.

According to Koens, the aim of any diet should be to form a safe, meaningful relationship with food, not to lose weight.

4. Low blood sugar

If you experience constant nausea, headaches, or dizziness while on the IF diet, it's a red flag that your blood sugar is out of whack. People with diabetes should avoid any form of fasting diet for this purpose, as stated by WH: Hypoglycemia, a risky condition for those with insulin or thyroid issues, may be caused by IF.

5. Hair loss

Is this for real? Yes. Hair loss can be caused by sudden weight loss or a lack of proper nutrients, especially protein and B vitamins, according to Koens.

Although intermittent fasting (IF) does not always result in nutritional loss, it is more difficult to eat a well-balanced diet when cramming a full day's worth of eating into a few hours. Reevaluate the nutrient quality of your daily meals and consult with your doctor about whether It is a good decision for you if you notice more hair falling out in the shower than normal.

6. Changes in your menstrual cycle

Another consequence of rapid weight loss (which may occur as a result of IF) is that women who lose a lot of weight or don't eat enough calories daily can notice that their menstrual cycles slow down or stop entirely.

What's With Intermittent Fasting On The Keto Diet?

According to the Mayo Clinic, people with unusually low body weight are vulnerable to amenorrhea or the lack of menstruation. Although you may be rejoicing about how IF has helped you lose pounds, you may still be depriving your body of the calories it needs to work.

If you're not having your period and suspect it's because of your intermittent fasting habits, stop fasting and talk to your gynecologist about it.

7. Constipation

Is it all backed up? It's possible that IF is to blame. "If you don't get enough fluid, vitamins, protein, or fiber, any diet can cause an upset stomach," says Koens, who stresses the importance of staying hydrated during the day.

People sometimes forget to drink water during fasting hours, but going 16 hours without enough fluid is a recipe for (gastrointestinal) disaster. So, if you've begun an IF diet and aren't having normal (or any) bowel movements, it's time to put your plan on hold and talk to a nutritionist or doctor about what's going on (or not going on in this case!).

8. Unhealthy diet

Even if IF does not cause a severe illness such as orthorexia, it may lead to poor eating behaviors. You can also find yourself making poor nutritional decisions during non-fasting hours and not having enough nutrients.

"The biggest concern is that you'll start binge-eating because you're so hungry," Charlie Seltzer, MD, a weight-loss physician and licensed personal trainer, previously told WH.

Can I Breastfeed While Intermittent Fasting?

If this describes you, you may benefit from working with an RD to develop a plan that doesn't require you to limit your eating hours and instead focuses on providing your body with the nutrients it needs every day, not just at those hours.

9. Sleep disturbances

Many people report better sleep patterns when doing IF, according to Koens, probably because IF helps curb late-night snacking behaviors, which can lead to an inability to fall asleep because your stomach is still digesting the 10 p.m. snack.

However, some evidence suggests that the opposite is true. Evidence suggests that intermittent diurnal fasting (daytime fasting) reduces rapid-eye-movement (REM) sleep, according to a study published in the journal Nature and Science of Sleep in 2018. According to the Harvard Business Review, getting enough REM sleep has been related to various health benefits, including improved memory, cognitive processing, and attention. It's unclear why this is the case.

If you're having trouble falling or staying asleep after starting an IF eating plan, pause and consult a professional to ensure you're not harming your health.

10. Mood changes

It'd be odd if you didn't have any moodiness throughout IF, at least at first. Although some people experience a significant increase in energy or motivation after adjusting to fasting, it's important to remember that it's still a restrictive diet. Feeling obliged to stick to it might make you depressed, particularly if you're isolating yourself from friends or family members due to your dietary restrictions.

Stop and speak with a licensed dietitian, counselor, or wellness coach right away if you're feeling down, nervous, or discouraged about IF. They may assist you in developing a fasting regimen that is more suitable for your mind and body.

This content was developed and maintained by a third party and was imported onto this website to assist users in entering their email addresses. You may be able to learn more about this and other related topics by visiting piano.

Refeeding syndrome

This extremely rare but life-threatening disorder can develop in underweight or malnourished people after a long fasting period.

These people can undergo potentially fatal changes in fluids and electrolytes during refeeding.

Most people who practice intermittent fasting will never have to think about this, which is one reason fasting is not recommended for underweight or malnourished people.

Who doesn't need to fast?

Intermittent fasting is not recommended for the following individuals.

1. Underweight or malnourished individuals: Fasting may deprive people underweight or malnourished of the nutrition and energy they need.

2. Someone who has had an eating disorder in the past (such as anorexia or bulimia): Fasting can cause certain disordered eating habits to resurface.

3. Children and adolescents: Since children and adolescents have higher growth demands, they need a constant supply of nutrition and energy. Without fasting, we suggest that overweight or obese children and adolescents concentrate on healthy eating habits.

4. Pregnant or breastfeeding women: Pregnancy and breastfeeding increase the mother's metabolic and nutritional needs, and fasting may lead to a failure to meet those needs.

5. Women trying to conceive: Fasting can cause a woman's body to ovulate irregularly or stop entirely, lowering her chances of becoming pregnant.

6. Those who think fasting causes them to binge eat, choose higher-carb foods, or consume more calories than they normally would: Some people don't have any contraindications to fasting. However, they find it causes them to binge eat, chooses higher-carb foods, or consume more calories than they normally would. This negates the benefits of fasting, so they can refrain from doing so.

Who needs special guidance?

Individuals who fall into the following categories may be able to fast successfully, but they should seek medical help from an experienced clinician to ensure their safety. Please contact us if you need assistance locating someone knowledgeable in this field.

Those who have diabetes and take medication: When fasting, anyone with type 1 or type 2 diabetes who takes blood-sugar-lowering drugs like insulin, sulfonylureas, and others may be at risk of dangerously low blood sugars. This is valid for both long and short-term fasts.

These people may still be able to fast, but they must be carefully coached and monitored by a trained professional.

1. People who take blood pressure medications: While the effect of fasting on blood pressure is less drastic than the effect on blood sugar, some people can find that their blood pressure drops too low when they fast. This is more of a problem with longer-term fasts but can also be a problem with shorter-term fasts. It's best to work under the supervision of a doctor.

2. Those who take other medications: Some medications, such as aspirin, ibuprofen, and other nonsteroidal anti-inflammatory drugs (NSAIDs), metformin, beta-blockers, and others, can cause digestive problems taken on an empty stomach.

If you're thinking of going on a short, don't forget to take your medications. It's important to first speak with your doctor about your choices for taking your drugs daily, missing them, or altering their timing.

3. People with serious medical conditions: Someone with a serious liver, kidney, heart or other medical condition may find it difficult to fast safely. Anyone suffering from one of these conditions should seek medical advice first.

How to break a fast

It's possible that how you break a fast is just as critical as the fast itself.

There are only a few items to remember for time-restricted eating (fasts of less than 24 hours) and short-term fasts (less than 36 hours):

1. Make sure you know what you're going to eat when you break your fast. When you're hungry and looking for something nutritious, the last thing you want to do when you're hungry and looking for something nutritious is shown up at a work function with pizza, bagels, and doughnuts.

2. Don't want to "make up" for lost calories. Remember that a normal decrease in calories is one of the advantages of time-restricted feeding. As if you hadn't fasted, eat your regular meals.

3. The only exception to the rule is that you will need to supplement your meals with a little extra protein to meet your regular goals.

CHAPTER 8: HOW CAN YOU INCORPORATE FASTING INTO YOUR EVERYDAY ROUTINE?

Despite the hundreds of "trendy" diet and weight loss books available on Amazon, changing your health does not have to be difficult. Take a minute to cleanse your mind of all the nonsense — keto this, gluten-free that. To improve your health, you don't need a 400-page diet book. Intermittent fasting can help you regain physiological balance, whether you're overweight, diabetic, or too busy for proper self-care. Intermittent fasting is gaining popularity as more people understand its value as a weight-loss and fitness hidden weapon.

After our first session about intermittent fasting, Zane Griggs and I realized we had much more to discuss, so he's back to delve deeper into this fascinating topic. If you're interested in intermittent fasting but don't know how to incorporate it into your daily routine, Zane, a professional fitness trainer, weight reduction coach, and intermittent fasting pioneer, is here to help.

What Characterizes a Successful Fast?

Is fasting simply avoiding meals? No, not at all.

"There are multiple ways to fast," Zane explains. In general, after around 12 hours of not eating any calories, our reliance on body fat for fuel increases." Intermittent fasting is defined as 12 hours between meals.

Your body mobilizes excess fat to burn energy after 12 hours. This means that going without food for a long time kickstarts weight reduction and produces a healthy gap that allows your body to regain homeostasis.

So, what constitutes a successful fast? Simply put, a good fast entails remaining out of your body for at least 12 hours. Successful fasting allows your body to reset, recalibrate, and burn fat rather than overfeeding it with food every few hours.

Intermittent fasting is most successful when a 14 to 18-hour period of minimal-calorie consumption is followed by a 10 to 6-hour period of good eating.

How to Begin Intermittent Fasting Some people can leap immediately into intermittent fasting, while others must gradually change their eating habits. I'm a member of that group! I was a food junkie, stumbling to the kitchen cabinet for breakfast before even getting out of bed, and it took me six months to learn how to fast occasionally.

We've been overfed as a country. This could take some time to adjust to eating less because we are conditioned to consume a large breakfast and snacks throughout the day. Perhaps you'll begin intermittent fasting on Mondays, Wednesdays, and Fridays, or just on weekends. Whatever method works best for you to get things started.

Every day, I speak with dedicated and disciplined patients in their employment, finances, beliefs, and relationships, but the food is the one roadblock they can't seem to overcome. Most other popular weight loss and wellness regimens have many difficulties and issues, but intermittent fasting does not.

It's simple to figure out how to master intermittent fasting and attain your goals without the fog of confusion.

Step 1: Skip Breakfast Zane, and I may have left your jaw on the floor during our last session when we discussed that the "advice" that breakfast is the most important meal of the day was established by a Grape-Nuts commercial.

The simplest and most effective approach to begin intermittent fasting is to eliminate breakfast from your daily routine. Your body does its miracle in the morning... In the morning, cortisol hormones and adrenals rise to help you wake up, become alert, and generate energy.

Why not make the most of your body's natural pattern to get the most out of fasting?

Step 2: When Is The Best Time To Workout? Believe they can't exercise while fasting; however, the contrary is true. The greatest time for a strong workout is in the morning! You're young and healthy, with hormonal balance on your side.

Afternoon and evening exercises aren't always as effective as they may be; you're tired from the day, distracted with whatever new pressures have been thrown in your path at work and battling the want to kick off your shoes and rest.

I stuck to my afternoon training regimen for over a decade, but switching to an early morning gym plan has been a game-changer. I can feel the sliding scale if I don't work out first thing in the morning since I lose my opportunity for a quality workout throughout the day. Life gets hectic, and the body becomes exhausted!

Step 3: Unwind. Your (unsweetened) coffee is still safe to drink!

"Can I drink coffee while fasting? "I know you're about to ask, your voice trembling.

"Yes! Fortunately for coffee enthusiasts everywhere, our beloved morning ritual does not raise blood sugar or cause a fast to be broken.

If you can't bear the idea of sipping black coffee, try adding some creamer. However, not too much! Remember that your body must burn through the fat in the creamer before it can return to burning your stored fat.

What about coffee consumers who need a sweetener to hide the bitterness? According to Zane, all-natural sweeteners such as cane sugar, honey, and agave nectar should be avoided. True, they're "natural" sugars, but they immediately spike blood sugar and insulin levels. Your body will no longer be in a fasting condition as a result.

Stick to a modest dash of Stevia in your coffee if you want a bit of sweetness. Most artificial sugars are harmful because they trigger cravings and deceive your digestive system into anticipating sugar that won't arrive. This messes with the fat-burning mechanism that fasting is supposed to help with.

In the end, the question of coffee comes down to your objectives. If you're trying to lose 50 pounds, adding cream to your morning coffee may stymie your efforts. On the other hand, a sweetened cup of coffee is far superior to a slice of cheesecake! It's all about striking the right balance.

Step 4. This is also for you, diabetics!

Zane works with diabetic customers regularly who believe intermittent fasting is too dangerous.

"I don't know of a better method to regulate diabetes or reverse those symptoms than finding a way to introduce fasting," he explains.

Type 2 diabetes is a blood sugar unbalance disease, and intermittent fasting is a potent strategy for decreasing and stabilizing blood sugar levels through improving eating habits.

Fasting, in my opinion, is the most effective tool my patients have for improving their glycemic control. If diabetics follow a purposeful, doctor-guided approach, they may be able to use fasting to remove their need for medication and decrease the complications of diabetes.

Step 5: Schedule Lunch And Dinner Using Fasting Rhythms You've heard enough; you're ready to enter the lovely world of intermittent fasting. So, when are you allowed to eat?

"The simplest approach...is to forgo breakfast and have coffee or tea instead," Zane explains. "If you want to lose weight, have a low-carb lunch and dinner." Your first meal of the day occurs after your fasting window has ended, which means you'll be eating for the next six to eight hours.

"It's a give-and-take situation. Make sure it fits into your schedule... It's fine if it takes six hours. Don't beat yourself up if it has to be nine one day," Zane emphasizes.

The beauty of intermittent fasting is that there is no right or wrong way to do it. It's one tool you can use to improve your health in whatever way works best for you.

Step 6: Join The Dinnertime Club There's a reason why most people skip breakfast in favor of dinner. Our evening meals are social and interpersonal. That's how it's been for millennia! We use dinner to unwind from the day, reconnect with family, and commemorate the passing of another day. You don't have to lose out on this once-in-a-lifetime opportunity.

Instead, use the time to develop mindfulness while eating. You'll appreciate every piece of your food far more than if you'd been nibbling all day.

Step 7: Eat for Your Purpose During intermittent fasting, we've defined when to open your mouth. But what should you consume once you've opened your mouth? There is no one-size-fits-all option; everything is dependent on your goals.

While you're fasting to lose weight, Zane suggests avoiding carbs and sugar. Preplan your daily meal to break your fast and make it as easy as possible for yourself. Having a full, low-carb lunch on hand will keep you from making hasty selections. Don't break your fast if Burger King is the only alternative.

Dinner should provide lean protein and a vegetable, although healthy starch or fat is also okay. Remember: You're rewarding yourself with nourishing, enjoyable foods, not punishing yourself!

Concentrate on real meals if you're fasting for health and longevity rather than weight loss. It would not be food now if it weren't food 100 years ago! Avoid processed, packaged foods and read labels to escape the hidden trap of added sugars. It's all about finding a good combination of proteins, healthy fats, and fruits and vegetables. You'll immediately control your consumption of those sneaky carbohydrates if you eat these genuine foods.

Step 8: Try a 24-hour fast once a week. Don't get too worked up over the 24-hour fast. Once you've gotten used to intermittent fasting, switching to a 24-hour fast once a week isn't such a big deal.

Starting a 24-hour fast after dinner is ideal. Instead of breaking your fast at 1:00 p.m. with lunch, wait a few hours and break it with dinner and celebration.

I know from experience how satisfying the first meal following a 24-hour fast is. It's unlike anything else. Not to mention the fat-burning and metabolic advantages of a 24-hour body reset.

Step 9: Say No to an Intermittent Fasting Cheat Day Zane doesn't mince words when it comes to cheating days: "I'm not even sure what the point is." For most individuals, a cheat day is similar to a binge day, but the consequences of the binge don't go away after 24 hours. It can take three or four days to recover from the impacts of a cheat day, reign in your desires, regain your energy and attention, and get back on track.

"Why throw it all off with a complete plate of pizza or a lot of pancakes if your aim is weight loss and you're trying to get there effectively?"

" Zane inquires. During an intermittent fasting cheat day, 1,500 junk food calories will push you away from your goals.

An indulgence, on the other hand, is a different matter. Itchy skin can be soothed with a piece of pie or some cookies now and then.

Fasting for Longevity Isn't Just About Losing Weight!

One of the essential health benefits of fasting is extending your body's time without direct energy sources. You don't have insulin if you raise your blood glucose levels for 16 or 18 hours. When you eventually eat anything that triggers an insulin response, the insulin appears, does its function, and then vanishes. Insulin sensitivity is the polar opposite of diabetes!

Fasting isn't about deprivation; it is about appreciating what you have. Instead of compulsively nibbling and suffering through your days in an overfed coma, you eat genuine meals when your body needs them.

In Zane's and my experience, intermittent fasting is the key to applying discipline to the art of eating. Intermediate fasting is feasible and doable for busy, highly successful people because it may be approached with defined goals and plans.

And, yeah, fasting is quite safe. You can keep a 16-hour intermittent fasting schedule daily and only benefit from it. Zane is a living example.

"I've been doing it every day for years!" I see fasting as a way to keep a healthy, active lifestyle into my 60s, 70s, and 80s." I couldn't agree with you more. Fasting, when broken down, is a technique to align your short-term goals, such as decreasing weight and increasing energy, with your long-term goals, such as postponing the onset of chronic diseases.

CHAPTER 9: RECIPES

1. ARM ROASTED VEGETABLE FARRO SALAD

Ready in: 1hr 35mins

Serves: 4

Yield: 4

INGREDIENTS

- One tablespoon kosher salt or One tablespoon sea salt
- 1/2 medium-sized eggplant, peel on, and large diced
- One cup cherry tomatoes washed and left whole
- Six white button mushrooms, quartered
- One medium-sized zucchini, peel on and large diced
- Six garlic cloves, peeled, trimmed, and sliced
- 1/2 medium-sized red onion, peeled and cut into wedges
- 1 cup cracked farro
- 2 cups almond milk (Almond Breeze)
- One tablespoon olive oil
- One teaspoon tbsp olive oil (15 mL)
- One tablespoon balsamic vinegar
- 3 sprigs fresh cilantro
- One tablespoon olive oil
- 1/2 teaspoon salt
- 1/2 teaspoon pepper

DIRECTIONS

1. Preheat the oven to 200 C (400 °F).
2. Salt the eggplant slices generously on all sides in a wide flat pan or baking sheet, toss to cover evenly, and keep for 30 minutes to release excess moisture and bitterness.
3. Drain the eggplant and rinse and toss it into a large mixing bowl. Tomatoes, zucchini, mushrooms, garlic, and onions are added. Drizzle the vegetables with olive oil generously, season with salt and pepper, and stir to coat. Move the vegetables to a pan lined with ovenproof tin foil. In the oven, roast the vegetables for 20 - 25 minutes or until tender, caramelized, and forked. To avoid sticking to the plate, stir or flip the vegetables about 10 to 15 minutes into the roasting process. Set aside and remove the pan from the oven.
4. Meanwhile, rinse the ferro with water and drain over the sink in a colander. Into a 3-quart (3L) saucepot, add the farro, and add in the Almond Breeze. A pinch of salt and a drizzle of olive oil is added. Bring the liquid to a boil over medium-high heat to prevent boiling, then turn the heat down to a gentle simmer. Simmer the farro with the lid on the pot cocked to one side for 20 minutes to let out steam. Turn off the heat but leave the pot and close

the lid on the stovetop. For another 5 minutes or until the farro is soft yet slightly chewy in the middle, steam in the pot. Using a fork to loosen the lid and the fluff.

5. Mix the cooked farro with the vegetables in a large serving dish and gently toss to mix until ready to assemble the dish. Whisk the balsamic vinegar along with the olive oil and drizzle over the farro salad. Toss to coat and season to taste with salt and pepper. Add fresh cilantro and a squeeze of lemon to garnish. Serve it sweet.

2. SHEET PAN CHICKEN AND BRUSSEL SPROUTS

Ready in: 40mins

Serves: 4

INGREDIENTS

- 1 1/2 cups Brussels sprouts, halved
- Four skin-on chicken thighs
- Four carrots, cut on the bias
- One teaspoon herbs de Provence
- Three tablespoons olive oil

DIRECTIONS

1. Preheat the stove to 400o F.
2. Put the cut vegetables in a bowl and add 11⁄2 tablespoons of olive oil, 1⁄2 tablespoons of herbs, salt, and pepper. Rub the vegetables all over.
3. On a sheet pan, place the veggies.
4. In the same bowl, add the chicken thighs. Drizzle with 11⁄2 tablespoons of olive oil, 1⁄2 tablespoons of herbs, salt, and pepper. Rub the chicken all over.
5. Put the chicken in a pan.
6. Roast for 30-35 minutes or until you're done with the chicken.
7. Turn the oven over to broil and cook for a minute or two if you prefer a crispier vegetable or chicken skin. Carefully watch, or it'll burn.

3. TRAIL MIX

Ready in: 2mins

Serves: 6

INGREDIENTS

- 1 cup sunflower seeds (raw)
- 1 cup almonds (raw)
- 1 cup raisins
- 1⁄4 cup flaked coconut (optional)
- 1⁄2 cup dried apricot (unsulphured, chopped)

- 1/4 cup carob chips (optional) or 1⁄4 cup chocolate (optional)

DIRECTIONS

1. Pour it all into a big container, cover it and shake it!
2. Store in a bag that is airtight. To preserve the properties of the essential fatty acids, place them in the fridge/freezer.

4. PERFECT CAULIFLOWER PIZZA CRUST

Ready in: 1hr 10mins

Serves: 4

INGREDIENTS

- One egg, beaten
- Four cups raw cauliflower, riced, or one medium cauliflower head
- One cup chevre cheese or 1 cup other soft cheese
- One pinch salt
- One teaspoon dried oregano

DIRECTIONS

1. Preheat to 400°F in your oven.
2. Pulse batches of raw cauliflower florets in a food processor to render the cauliflower rice until a rice-like texture are achieved.

3. Fill a big pot and bring it to a boil with around an inch of water. Connect the "rice" and cover; cook for 5 minutes or so. Drain the strainer into a fine-mesh one.

4. THIS IS THE SECRET: Move it to a clean, thin dishtowel once you've strained the rice. In the dishtowel, cover the steamed rice, curl it and Suck out all the excess moisture! It's amazing how much extra liquid will be released, leaving you with a good dry crust of the pizza.

5. Mix your strained rice, beaten egg, goat's cheese, and spices in a big bowl. (Don't fear using your hands! You want it mixed well.) It's not going to be like every pizza dough you've ever dealt with, yet don't worry, it's going to stay together!

6. On a baking sheet lined with parchment paper, press the dough out. Keep the dough about 3/8" thick, and make the edges a little higher for a "crust" effect, if you like. (It must be lined with parchment paper, or it will stick.)"

7. Bake at 400 ° F for 35-40 minutes. The crust should be firm and, when done, golden brown.

8. Now's the time to add sauce, cheese, and any other toppings you want to all your favorites. Put the pizza back in the oven for 400F and bake for an additional 5-10 minutes, only until the cheese is hot and bubbly.

9. Cut and quickly serve!

5. CAJUN POTATO, PRAWN/SHRIMP AND AVOCADO SALAD

Ready in: 30mins

Serves: 2

INGREDIENTS

- One tablespoon olive oil
- 300 g new potatoes (small baby or chats 10 oz halved)
- 250 g king prawns (8 oz, cooked and peeled)
- Two spring onions (finely sliced)
- One garlic clove (minced)
- Two teaspoons cajun seasoning
- 1 cup alfalfa sprout
- 1avocado (peeled, stoned, and diced)
- salt (to boil potatoes)

DIRECTIONS

1. Cook the potatoes for 10 to 15 minutes in a large saucepan of lightly salted boiling water, or until tender, then drain well.

2. In a wok or a large nonstick frying pan/skillet, heat the oil.
3. Season with the prawns, garlic, spring onions, and cajun and fry for 2 to 3 minutes or until the prawns are hot.
4. Stir in the potatoes, then cook for an additional minute.
5. Transfer to dishes for serving and top with the avocado and sprouts of alfalfa and eat.

6. BAKED MAHI MAHI

Ready in: 40mins

Serves: 4

INGREDIENTS

- 2 lbs mahi-mahi (4 fillets)
- 1/4 teaspoon garlic salt
- One lemon, juiced
- 1 cup mayonnaise
- 1/4 cup white onion, finely chopped
- 1/4 teaspoon ground black pepper
- breadcrumbs

DIRECTIONS

1. Preheat the oven to 425 degrees.
2. Put it in a baking dish and rinse the fish. Squeeze the fish with lemon juice and sprinkle with garlic, salt, and pepper.
3. Combine the mayonnaise and the chopped onions and scatter them over the fish. Sprinkle with breadcrumbs and bake for 25 minutes at 425°F.

7. SWEET POTATO AND BLACK BEAN BURRITO

Ready in: 1hr 5mins

Yield: 8-12 portions

INGREDIENTS

- 5 cups peeled cubed sweet potatoes
- two teaspoons other vegetable oil or two teaspoons broth
- 1/2 teaspoon salt
- 3 1/2 cups diced onions
- One tablespoon minced fresh green chili pepper
- 4garlic cloves, minced (or pressed)
- Four teaspoons ground cumin
- 4 1/2 cups cooked black beans (three 15-ounce cans, drained)
- Four teaspoons ground coriander

- 2/3 cup lightly packed cilantro leaf
- One teaspoon salt
- 12 (10 inches) flour tortillas
- Two tablespoons fresh lemon juice
- fresh salsa

DIRECTIONS

1. preheat the oven To 350*.
2. Place the salt and water in a medium saucepan to cover the sweet potatoes.
3. Cover and bring to a boil, then simmer for about 10 minutes, until tender.
4. Drain yourself and set aside.
5. Heat the oil in a medium saucepan or skillet while the sweet potatoes are frying, and add the onions, garlic, and chili.
6. On medium-low heat, cover and cook, occasionally stirring, until the onions are tender, around 7 minutes.
7. Add cumin and coriander and cook, constantly stirring, for 2 to 3 minutes longer.
8. Remove and set aside from the sun.
9. Combine the black beans, lemon juice, cilantro, salt, and cooked sweet potatoes in a food processor and puree until smooth (or mash the ingredients in a large bowl by hand).

10. In a large mixing bowl, pass the sweet potato mixture and blend in the cooked onions and spices.
11. Oil a large baking dish lightly.
12. At the center of each tortilla, spoon around 2/3 to 3/4 cup of the filling, roll it up, and put it in the baking dish, seam side down.
13. Cover thoroughly with foil and bake for 30 minutes or so, until sweet.
14. Serve with salsa topping.

8. SWEET POTATO CURRY WITH SPINACH AND CHICKPEAS

Ready in: 30mins

Serves: 6

INGREDIENTS

- 1 -2 teaspoon canola oil
- One tablespoon cumin
- Two tablespoons curry powder
- One teaspoon cinnamon
- 1⁄2 large sweet onions, chopped or two scallions, thinly sliced
- ten ounces fresh spinach washed, stemmed, and coarsely chopped

- One (14 1/2 ounce) can chickpeas, rinsed and drained
- Two large sweet potatoes, peeled and diced (about 2 lbs)
- 1/2 cup water
- 1/4 cup chopped fresh cilantro for garnish
- One (14 1/2 ounce) can diced tomatoes, can substitute fresh if available
- basmati rice or brown rice, for serving

DIRECTIONS

1. Whatever you like, you can choose to cook sweet potatoes.
2. I enjoy peeling, slicing, and steaming mine for about 15 minutes in a veggie steamer.
3. Fit well baking or boiling, too.
4. Heat 1-2 tsp of canola or vegetable oil over medium heat while the sweet potatoes are cooking.
5. Add the onions and sauté for three minutes, or until tender.
6. Add the curry powder, cumin, and cinnamon, then stir to cover the spices' onions evenly.
7. Stir in the tomatoes and their juices, and stir in the chickpeas to blend.
8. Add half a cup of water and lift the heat for about a minute or two to a high simmer.

9. Then add fresh spinach, stirring to cover with cooking liquid, a few handfuls at a time.

10. Cover and boil until just wilted, about 3 minutes, when all the spinach is added to the pan.

11. Apply to the liquid the cooked sweet potatoes, and stir to coat.

12. Simmer for another five minutes, or until you mix the flavors well.

13. Move to a dish for serving, toss with fresh cilantro and serve sweet.

14. This dish is served beautifully over basmati or brown rice.

9. CROCKPOT BLACK EYED PEAS

Ready in: 10hrs 5mins

Serves: 6

INGREDIENTS

- One small ham hock
- 1 (16 ounces) bag dried black-eyed peas
- One (14 1/2 ounce) can diced tomatoes with green chilies
- One (14 1/2 ounce) can Del Monte zesty jalapeno pepper diced tomato
- One stalk celery, chopped

- Two (10 1/2 ounce) can chicken broth

DIRECTIONS

1. Following the directions on the bag, pre-soak black-eyed peas.
2. Combine all ingredients and cook for 9-10 hours on low heat.

10. PEACH BERRY SMOOTHIE

Ready in: 5mins

Serves: 1

INGREDIENTS

- One cup frozen peaches
- 1/2 cup Greek yogurt
- 1/4 cup coconut milk (adjust for a thicker or thinner smoothie)
- 1/2 teaspoon almond flavoring

DIRECTIONS

1. In a high-speed blender, blend the peaches with almond flavoring.
2. Check and change the thickness accordingly. For thinner, add more milk, and for thicker, more peaches.

3. Gorgeous toppings such as chia seeds, berries, and slivered almonds are on top.

11. SHREDDED BRUSSELS SPROUTS WITH BACON AND ONIONS

Ready in: 30mins

Serves: 6

INGREDIENTS

- One small yellow onion, thinly sliced
- Two slices of bacon
- 3⁄4 cup water
- One teaspoon Dijon mustard
- 1⁄4 teaspoon salt (or to taste)
- One tablespoon cider vinegar
- 1 lb Brussels sprout, trimmed, halved, and very thinly sliced

DIRECTIONS

1. Cook bacon in a big pan until crisp (5 to 7 minutes) over medium heat; drain on paper towels, then crumble.

2. Transfer the onion and salt to the pan's drippings and cook over medium heat until tender and browned, frequently stirring (about 3 minutes).
3. Add water and mustard, scrape any browned parts, add sprouts from Brussels and cook, stirring regularly, until tender (4 to 6 minutes).
4. Stir in the vinegar and add the crumbled bacon to the tip.

12. MAMA'S SUPPER CLUB TILAPIA PARMESAN

Ready in: 35mins

Serves: 4

INGREDIENTS

- 1/2 cup grated parmesan cheese
- Two tablespoons lemon juice
- Three tablespoons mayonnaise
- Three tablespoons finely chopped green onions
- Four tablespoons butter, room temperature
- 1/4 teaspoon dried basil
- black pepper
- 1/4 teaspoon seasoning salt (I like Old Bay seasoning here)
- One dash of hot pepper sauce
- 2 lbs tilapia fillets (orange roughy, cod, or red snapper can be substituted)

DIRECTIONS

1. Preheat the oven to 350°C.
2. Lay the fillets in a single layer in a buttered 13-by-9-inch baking dish or jelly roll pan.
3. Do not have fillets stacked.
4. Brush with juice on top.
5. Mix the cheese, butter, mayonnaise, onions, and seasonings in a dish.
6. Blend well with the fork.
7. In a preheated oven, bake the fish for 10 to 20 minutes or until the fish just begins to flake.
8. Spread with cheese mixture and bake for around 5 minutes, until golden brown.
9. Baking time will depend on the fish thickness that you are using.
10. Control the fish carefully so that they do not overcook.
11. Note: You can make this fish in a broiler, too.
12. Broil for 3-4 minutes or until nearly through.
13. Attach the cheese and broil for 2 to 3 minutes or until it is browned.

13. ROASTED BROCCOLI W LEMON GARLIC AND TOASTED PINE NUTS

Ready in: 22mins

Serves: 4

INGREDIENTS

- 1 lb broccoli floret
- salt & freshly ground black pepper
- Two tablespoons olive oil
- Two tablespoons unsalted butter
- 1/2 teaspoon lemon zest, grated
- One teaspoon garlic, minced
- 1 -2 tablespoon fresh lemon juice
- Two tablespoons pine nuts, toasted

DIRECTIONS

1. Preheat the oven to 500°C.
2. Toss the broccoli with the oil in a wide bowl and add salt and pepper to taste.
3. On a baking sheet, arrange the florets into a single layer and roast, turning once for 12 minutes or until just tender.
4. Melt the butter in a saucepan over medium heat.
5. Apply the zest of garlic and lemon and heat for about 1 minute, stirring.
6. Let the lemon juice cool slightly and stir it in.
7. Put the broccoli in a serving bowl, pour the lemon butter over it, and toss to coat it.
8. Scatter the toasted pine nuts over the top.

14. BEST BAKED POTATO

Ready in: 1hr 10mins

Serves: 1

INGREDIENTS

- canola oil
- One large russet potato
- kosher salt

DIRECTIONS

1. Heat the oven to 350 ° F and place the upper and lower thirds of the racks.
2. Thoroughly wash the potato (or potatoes) with a stiff brush and co1ld running water.
3. Dry, then poke 8 to 12 deep holes all over the spud using a regular fork so that moisture can escape during cooking.
4. Place it in a bowl and gently coat it with oil.
5. Sprinkle with kosher salt and put the potato in the middle of the oven directly on a rack.
6. To trap any drippings, place a baking sheet (I placed a piece of aluminum foil) on the lower rack.

7. Bake until the skin feels crisp, but the flesh feels soft underneath.
8. Serve by forming a dotted line with your fork from end to end, then crack the spud open by pressing the ends towards each other.
9. It's going to pop open right.
10. But watch out, there's going to be some steam there.

You will need to increase the cooking time by up to 15 minutes if you are cooking more than four potatoes.

15. EASY BLACK BEAN SOUP

Ready in: 25mins

Serves: 4

INGREDIENTS

- Three tablespoons olive oil
- one tablespoon ground cumin
- One medium onion, chopped
- 2 -3 cloves garlic
- two (14 1/2 ounce) cans of black beans
- salt and pepper
- two cups chicken broth or 2 cups vegetable broth
- One small red onion, chopped fine
- 1/4 cup cilantro, coarsely chopped or finely chopped (whatever you prefer)

DIRECTIONS

1. In olive oil, saute the onion.
2. Add cumin when the onion becomes translucent.
3. Cook for 30 seconds, add garlic, and cook for an additional 30 to 60 seconds.
4. Add one can of vegetable broth and 2 cups of black beans.
5. Bring to a boil, sometimes stirring.
6. Turn the heat off.
7. Mix the ingredients in the pot using a hand blender, or switch them to a blender.
8. Connect the second can of beans and the mixed ingredients to the pot and bring to a simmer.
9. Serve the soup with red onion bowls and cilantro for garnishing.
10. I'm also adding a bit of cilantro to the pot.
11. It can be doubled or frozen.

16. CAULIFLOWER POPCORN ROASTED CAULIFLOWER

Ready in: 1hr 10mins

Serves: 4

INGREDIENTS

- Four tablespoons olive oil
- one head cauliflower or one equal head amount of pre-cut commercially prepped cauliflower
- one teaspoon salt, to taste

DIRECTIONS

1. Preheat the oven to 425°C.
2. Trim the cauliflower head, discarding the thick stems and the core; cut the florets into pieces around the ping-pong balls' size.
3. Combine the olive oil and salt in a large bowl, whisk, then add the pieces of cauliflower and toss thoroughly.
4. For quick cleaning, line a baking sheet with parchment (you can skip that, if you don't have one, then spread the cauliflower pieces on the sheet and roast for 1 hour, turning three or four times, until most of each piece turns golden brown.
5. (The browner the pieces of cauliflower turn, the more caramelization happens and the sweeter they taste).
6. Serve and drink it instantly!

17. VEGAN LENTIL BURGERS

Ready in: 1hr 10mins

Yield: 8-10 burgers

INGREDIENTS

- 2 1⁄2 cups water
- 1 cup dry lentils, well rinsed
- 1⁄2 teaspoon salt
- 1⁄2 medium onion, diced
- One carrot, diced
- One tablespoon olive oil
- One teaspoon pepper
- One tablespoon soy sauce
- 3⁄4 cup breadcrumbs
- 3⁄4 cup rolled oats, finely ground

DIRECTIONS

1. Boil the lentils with the salt in the water for about 45 minutes. The lentils are going to be soft, and much of the water is gone.
2. It will take about five minutes to fry the onions and carrots in oil until tender.
3. The cooked ingredients are combined in a bowl with pepper, soy sauce, oats, and bread crumbs.
4. While the mixture is still warm, it will produce ten burgers.
5. Burgers can then be fried shallowly on each side for 1-2 minutes or baked for 15 minutes at 200C.

18. SAUERKRAUT SALAD

Ready in: 15mins

Serves: 6

INGREDIENTS

- 1 cup celery, chopped fine
- 1 (1 lb) can sauerkraut, drained but not rinsed
- 1/2 cup green pepper, chopped fine
- 1/2 teaspoon salt
- Two tablespoons onions, chopped fine
- 1/2 teaspoon pepper
- 1/3 cup salad oil
- 3/4 cup sugar
- 1/3 cup cider (I use white) or 1/3 cup white vinegar (I use white)

DIRECTIONS

1. Mix the sauerkraut with the chopped vegetables.
2. On low heat, heat the sugar, oil, vinegar, salt, and pepper until the sugar dissolves.
3. Refrigerate and pour over the vegetables.
4. Overnight relax.

19. VEGAN COCONUT KEFIR BANANA MUFFINS

Ready in: 45mins

Serves: 12

INGREDIENTS

- 2 cups all-purpose flour
- 1 cup unsweetened dried shredded coconut
- 1 cup granulated sugar
- Two teaspoons baking soda
- 1/2 teaspoon salt
- Two ripe bananas, mashed
- One teaspoon baking powder
- 1/4 cup cold-pressed liquid coconut oil
- 1 1/2 cups pc dairy-free kefir probiotic fermented coconut milk
- one teaspoon vanilla extract

DIRECTIONS

1. Preheat the oven to 180oC (350oF). Mist 12-Count Cooking Spray Muffin Tin. Only set aside.

2. In a big bowl, whisk together the flour, sugar, coconut, baking soda, baking powder, and salt. Only set aside.

3. In a separate, large cup, whisk together the bananas, kefir, coconut oil, and vanilla. Add to the flour mixture; stir until there are no white streaks left.

4. Divide the prepared muffin tin between the wells. Cook until the tops are golden and the toothpick inserted in the

centers comes out clean, about 30 minutes. Let it cool for fifteen minutes in the muffin pan.

Chef's tip: let them cool fully on a rack to freeze muffins, then move to an airtight container and freeze for up to a month. You may individually cover the muffins in plastic wrap or foil before placing them in the container or bag for additional protection against freezer burn. In the oven, Overnight thaw muffins or microwave straight from frozen until warmed through around 20 to 30 seconds.

20. BERRY CRISP - WEIGHT WATCHERS CORE RECIPE

Ready in: 45mins

Serves: 6

INGREDIENTS

FRUIT

- 1 (7/8 ounce) box jello sugar-free vanilla pudding mix, cook and serve
- 1/2 teaspoon nutmeg
- 1 (16 ounces) bag cherries or (16 ounces) bag blueberries
- 1/4 cup nonfat milk

- One teaspoon cinnamon

CRISP

- 1 1/2 cups old fashioned oats
- 8 ounces plain fat-free yogurt
- One teaspoon almond extract
- 1/2 cup Splenda sugar substitute

DIRECTIONS

1. Spray an 8X8 baking pan.
2. In the pan, mix up the fruit ingredients and stir well.
3. Mix the crisp mixture in a separate dish.
4. To make a top crust, extend this mixture over the berry mixture.
5. Bake for 40-45 minutes at 350 F or until the top becomes crunchy.

21. ZUCCHINI AND EGGS RECIPE WITH CHEESE

Cook Time: 16 minutes

Prep Time: 4 minutes

Total Time: 20 minutes

Servings: 1 serving

INGREDIENTS

- One yellow onion small, sliced thinly, about 4 ounces
- One tablespoon olive oil separated
- 2-3 garlic cloves sliced in half
- One small zucchini chopped into ½-inch quarters (see note), about 6 ounces
- One egg room temperature, slightly beaten
- salt and pepper to taste
- One tablespoon water
- One tablespoon Italian parsley chopped
- 1-2 tablespoons Romano cheese grated

INSTRUCTIONS

1. Heat 1⁄2 tablespoons of olive oil over medium-high heat in a large skillet.
2. Add the onion and reduce to medium heat.
3. Cook, stirring until translucent periodically and softened for around 3-5 minutes.
4. The remaining chopped zucchini, olive oil, and garlic are added. With salt and pepper, season.
5. Saute, stirring and shaking the pan, until golden brown, over medium-high heat. It should take about 7-10 minutes for this. The zucchini needs to be baked, but it's still crisp—taste of doneness. If necessary, change the heat.
6. Meanwhile, whisk the cheese and parsley with the egg.

7. Add the egg mixture to the pan when the zucchini is cooked, and let it cook for about 30 seconds. Then stir and shake the pan until the egg is scrambled and set for 1 minute or so.
8. Taste the seasonings and change.
9. Immediately serve.
10. Garnish with chopped Italian parsley and grated cheese, if needed.

Nutrition

Serving: 1serving | Carbohydrates: 17g | Calories: 280kcal | Protein: 10g | Fat: 20g | Saturated Fat: 4g | Sodium: 141mg | Potassium: 529mg | Cholesterol: 169mg | Fiber: 3g | Sugar: 8g | Iron: 2mg Vitamin A: 811IU | Vitamin C: 36mg | Calcium: 133mg |

22. SPICY SPANISH TOMATO BAKED EGGS

INGREDIENTS

- One tbsp olive oil
- One red pepper, deseeded and cut into strips
- Two red onions, peeled and cut into half-moons
- One clove garlic, peeled and sliced
- 1 tsp paprika

- Four medium eggs
- 250g cherry tomatoes, halved or one tin peeled plum tomatoes
- Two tbsp chopped flat-leaf parsley (optional)

METHOD

1. Preheat the oven to 180 ° C/Gas 6 200 ° C/fan
2. Heat the oil in a large, deep, ovenproof frying pan,
3. Add the onions, garlic, and pepper. Season with freshly ground black pepper and cook until soft or for 10 minutes.
4. Add the tomatoes and paprika and cook gently for an additional 5 minutes.
5. In the mixture, make four little wells and crack an egg into each. Season, cover, and place in the oven with black pepper.
6. Cook until the eggs are set - this should take 5-8 minutes or so. If used, sprinkle over the parsley.

23. EGG SCRAMBLE WITH SWEET POTATOES

INGREDIENTS:

- ½ cup chopped onion
- 1 (8-oz) sweet potato, diced
- 2 tsp chopped rosemary
- Salt

- Four large eggs
- Four large egg whites
- Pepper
- 2 tbsp chopped chive

DIRECTIONS:

1. Preheat the heater to 425 degrees F. Toss the sweet potato, onion, rosemary, salt, and pepper on a baking dish. Spray with cooking spray and roast for about 20 minutes, until tender.
2. Meanwhile, whisk the eggs, egg whites, and a pinch of salt and pepper together in a medium cup. Spritz a cooking spray skillet and scramble the eggs over medium heat for around 5 minutes.
3. Sprinkle and serve with the spuds with chopped chives.
4. 571 calories per serving, 44 g of protein, 52 g of carbohydrates (9 g of fibre), 20 g of fat

24. ITALIAN CHICKEN

Cook Time30 minutes

Prep Time10 minutes

Total Time40 minutes

INGREDIENTS

- Four boneless skinless chicken breasts
- 1/2 cup breadcrumbs
- 1/2 cup grated parmesan cheese
- 1/2 teaspoon minced garlic
- salt and pepper to taste
- Four tablespoons butter melted
- One teaspoon Italian seasoning
- 1 pound small potatoes halved or quartered
- cooking spray
- Two tablespoons chopped parsley
- lemon wedges optional garnish

INSTRUCTIONS

1. To 400 degrees, preheat the oven. Using cooking spray to cover a sheet pan.
2. Mix the parmesan cheese, breadcrumbs, garlic, Italian seasoning, salt, and pepper in a small cup.
3. In the melted butter, dip the top of each chicken breast, then press the chicken's top into the breadcrumb mixture to coat it.
4. On the prepared sheet pan, put the chicken breasts.
5. About the chicken, scatter the potatoes. Drizzle over the potatoes and chicken with the remaining butter. With salt and pepper, season the potatoes.

6. Bake for thirty minutes or until the chicken is completely cooked and the potatoes are tender. The cooking time can vary depending on the thickness of your chicken.
7. Sprinkle and serve with parsley. If needed, garnish with lemon wedges.

NUTRITION

Carbohydrates: 10g | Calories: 336kcal |

Protein: 30g | Fat: 18g | Saturated

Fat: 10g | Cholesterol: 113mg | Vitamin A: 490IU |

Potassium: 460mg | Vitamin C: 1.3mg | Sodium:

520mg | Calcium: 172mg | Iron: 1.2mg

25. ORIENTAL TURKEY BURGERS

INGREDIENTS

SLAW

- 2 cups coleslaw mix
- One tablespoon seasoned rice vinegar
- Three tablespoons chopped fresh cilantro
- One teaspoon vegetable oil

BURGER

- Two tablespoons Butter
- Two jalapeño chile peppers, seeded, finely chopped
- 1/3 cup chopped green onions
- 1 1/4 pounds lean ground turkey
- One tablespoon hoisin sauce
- One tablespoon soy sauce
- 1/4 cup dry bread crumbs
- One tablespoon butter, melted
- Hoisin sauce, if desired
- 5 (10-inch) tortillas

DIRECTIONS

1. heat the gas grill until the coals are ash white on a medium or charcoal grill.
2. In a tub, mix all the slaw ingredients; mix well. Cover; leave to cool before serving time.
3. Melt two tablespoons of butter until sizzling in a 10-inch skillet; add the onion and chili peppers. Cook for approximately 1-2 minutes or until tender. Cool.
4. In a cup, combine the onion mix, turkey, bread crumbs, one tablespoon of hoisin sauce, and soy sauce; mix gently. Shape into four patties (3/4 inches thick).
5. Set the patties on the grill—a molten butter brush. Grill, rotating once, 20-30 minutes or until the

inner temperature reaches a minimum of 165 °f and the middle of the meat is no longer pink.

6. Wrap the aluminum foil tortillas. Place them away from direct heat on the grill. Move tortillas often when grilling burgers.

7. Place half of each warm tortilla with the burgers. Top with slaw; drizzle, if necessary, with hoisin sauce. Fold your tortilla over your burger.

26. VEGETABLE MEATLOAF WITH BALSAMIC GLAZE

INGREDIENTS

- Two tablespoons extra-virgin olive oil
- One small zucchini, finely diced
- One large egg, lightly beaten
- One red bell pepper, finely diced
- One yellow bell pepper, finely diced
- Five cloves garlic smashed to a paste with coarse salt
- Kosher salt and freshly ground pepper
- 1/4 cup chopped fresh parsley
- 1/2 cup Parmesan cheese or freshly grated Romano
- 1 1/2 pounds ground turkey (90% lean)
- 1 cup panko (coarse Japanese breadcrumbs)
- One tablespoon finely chopped fresh thyme
- 1/4 cup plus two tablespoons balsamic vinegar

- 3/4 cup ketchup

DIRECTIONS

1. The oven should be preheated to 425 degrees. Over high pressure, heat the oil in a large saute pan. Add the zucchini, garlic paste, bell peppers, and 1/4 teaspoon of red pepper flakes. Season with pepper and salt and cook for about 5 minutes, until the vegetables are almost tender. Set to cool aside.

2. In a large cup, whisk in the egg and fresh herbs. Add turkey, panko, grated cheese, 1/2 cup of ketchup, two tablespoons of cooled vegetables, and balsamic vinegar; blend until just mixed.

3. Press the mixture into a 9-by-5-inch loaf pan gently. In a small bowl, whisk the remaining 1/4 cup balsamic vinegar and1/4 cup ketchup, 1/4 teaspoon red pepper flakes; brush the blend over the whole loaf. For 1 to 1 1/4 hours, bake. Until slicing, let it rest for 10 minutes.

27. BUFFALO CHICKEN SANDWICH WITH BLUE CHEESE SLAW

INGREDIENTS

Blue Cheese Slaw:

- 1/4 cup mayonnaise

- One tablespoon minced garlic
- 1/4 cup crumbled blue cheese
- Two tablespoons Worcestershire sauce
- 1 (10-ounce) package coleslaw mix
- Kosher salt
- One lemon, juiced
- Freshly cracked black pepper
- Canola oil, to fry

Buffalo Chicken:

- 1/2 cup buffalo hot sauce, store-bought
- Two tablespoons smoked paprika, plus more for seasoning
- 4 (6-ounce) boneless, skinless chicken cutlets
- One tablespoon kosher salt, plus more for seasoning
- One cup self-rising flour
- 1 1/4 cups buttermilk
- Two tablespoons hot sauce
- One egg
- One tablespoon cracked black pepper, plus more for seasoning
- Four soft-club rolls, split and toasted

DIRECTIONS

1. Mix the mayonnaise, crumbled blue cheese, garlic, Worcestershire sauce, and lemon juice in a medium-sized bowl until well mixed. Attach the mix of

coleslaw and toss well. With salt and pepper, season and set aside.

2. Heat enough canola oil in a deep-fryer or heavy-bottomed pot to get halfway up the sides of the pot to 350 degrees F.

3. In a shallow dish, add buffalo sauce and set aside. To taste, season the chicken with smoked paprika and salt and pepper. In a shallow dish, place the flour, two tablespoons of paprika, one tablespoon of salt, and one tablespoon of pepper. Put the egg, buttermilk, and hot sauce together in another shallow dish and whisk together. Dredge each piece of chicken, shake off any excess in the buttermilk mixture, and then dredge it into the flour mixture. Fry until the chicken is cooked for around 4 to 6 minutes. On an instant-read thermometer, the internal temperature registers 165 degrees F. In the buffalo sauce, dip the finished chicken and place it on the club rolls. Top the chicken and shape a sandwich with a liberal quantity of slaw.

28. EASY BBQ CHICKEN TOSTADAS

Prep Time10 mins

Total Time18 mins

Cook Time8 mins

Servings: 4

INGREDIENTS

- Three cups cooked and shredded chicken
- One 1/2 cups of your favorite barbecue sauce, divided
- Eight tostada shells or eight corn tortillas brushed lightly with olive oil and baked for 3-5 minutes per side, until crispy
- Three green onions, very thinly sliced (optional)
- Two cups shredded cheese (Mary uses mozzarella in the cookbook, but I have also used cheddar, Monterey Jack, or a blend)

INSTRUCTIONS

1. Preheat to 350°F in your oven. Spread out two rimmed baking sheets with the tostada shells (or baked tortillas).
2. In a small bowl, mix the chicken and 1 cup barbecue sauce, and swirl to coat.
3. Divide the chicken between the shells of the tostada and top with the cheese (approximately 1/4 cup each).
4. Bake, only until the cheese is melted, for 6 to 8 minutes.

5. Remove and drizzle with the remaining 1/2 cup of barbecue sauce from the oven. If needed, sprinkle it with green onions.

Nutrition

Serving: 2tostadas | Vitamin A: 825IU | Calories: 693kcal | Carbohydrates: 66g | Protein: 31g | Fat: 33g | Saturated Fat: 13g | Sodium: 1730mg | Potassium: 554mg | Fiber: 3g | Sugar: 36g | Vitamin C: 3.7mg | Calcium: 359mg | Cholesterol: 107mg | Iron: 2.3mg

CHAPTER 10: 21-DAY MEAL PLAN

16/8 PLAN

WEEK 1

DAY 1

8: 00am: Warm Lemon Honey Water

11:00 am - Breakfast: ½ Chees/Bagel/Egg/Coconut Cream/Coffee

3:00 pm - Snack: Kind Bar

5:00 pm - Diner: Green Beans with Sauteed Chicken Breast

Brown Rice

7:00 pm – Fasting

DAY 2

8:00 am: Warm Lemon Honey Water

11:00 am - BREAKFAST: Coconut Creamer/Greek Yogurt/Coffee

3:00 pm - SNACK: Apple Slices

140

5:00 pm - DINNER: Steamed Broccoli, Grilled Salmon, Brown Rice

7:00 pm - Fasting

DAY 3

8:00 am: Warm Lemon Honey Water

11:00 am - BREAKFAST: Almond Butter/Oatmeal

Coffee/Coconut Creamer

3:00 pm - SNACK: Nuts

5:00 pm - DINNER: Tomatoes/Sauteed Egg

Brown Rice

7:00 pm: Fasting

DAY 4

8:00 am – Warm Lemon Honey Water

11:00 am – BREAKFAST: Coconut Creamer/Coffee

Avocado Toast/Egg

3:00 pm – SNACK: Banana/Strawberry Smoothie

5:00 pm – DINNER: Steamed Broccoli

Teriyaki Chicken

Brown Rice

7:00 pm – Fasting

DAY 5

8:00 am – Warm Lemon Honey Water

11:00 am – BREAKFAST: Triple Berry Smoothies

Coconut Creamer/Coffee

3:00 pm – SNACK: Nuts

5:00 pm – DINNER: Cauliflower Rice with Sauteed Chicken and Mushroom

7:00 pm- Fasting

DAY 6

8:00 am – Warm Lemon Honey Water

11:00 am – BREAKFAST: Whole Wheat Pancake

Coconut Creamer/Coffee

3:00 pm – SNACK: Blueberries

5:00 pm – DINNER: Dine Out

7:00 pm – Fasting

DAY 7

8:00 am – Warm Lemon Honey Water

9:00 am – Coconut Milk with Coffee

11:00 am – Breakfast Skip

3:00 ppm – SNACK: Nuts

5:00 pm - DINNER: Ground Pork and Spinach with Soba

Noodle

7:00 pm: Fasting

WEEK 2

DAY 8

8:00 am: Lemon water

8:30 am: Skip breakfast

12:00 pm: Avocado chicken salad

3:00 pm: Nuts

7:00 pm: Macadamia basil pesto pasta

8:00 pm: Begin fasting

DAY 9

8:00 am: Black coffee

8:30 am: Skip breakfast

12:00 pm: Vegan chickpea salad

3:00 pm: Fruit of your choice

7:00 pm: Mexican tempeh

8:00 pm: Begin fasting

DAY 10

8:00 am: Black coffee

8:30 am: Skip breakfast

12:00 pm: Tuna avocado salad wrap

3:00 pm: Hummus & raw veggie sticks

7:00 pm: Asian fried noodles

8:00 pm: Begin fasting

DAY 11

8:00 am: Apple cider vinegar drink

8:30 am: Skip breakfast

12:00 pm: Broccoli tofu salad

3:00 pm: Dark chocolate

7:00 pm: Salmon kale salad

8:00 pm: Begin fasting

DAY 12

8:00 am: Lemon water

8:30 am: Skip breakfast

12:00 pm: Turkey chili

3:00 pm: Organic edamamae

7:00 pm: Grilled chicken salad

8:00 pm: Begin fasting

DAY 13

8:00 am: Lemon water

8:30 am: Skip breakfast

12:00 pm: Grilled salmon

3:00 pm: Dark chocolate bark

7:00 pm: Chicken tortilla soup

8:00 pm: Begin fasting

DAY 14

8: 00 am: Black coffee

8:30 am: Skip breakfast

12:00 pm: Sprouts, chicken, quinoa Buddah bowl

3:00 pm: Greek yogurt

7:00 pm: Teriyaki chicken with cauliflower rice

8:00 pm: Begin fasting

WEEK 3

DAY 15

8:00 am: Lemon water

8:30 am: Skip breakfast

12:00 pm: Grilled salmon

3:00 pm: Dark chocolate bark

7:00 pm: Chicken tortilla soup

8:00 pm: Begin fasting

DAY 16

8:00 am: Black coffee

8:30 am: Skip

12:00 pm: Mexican chicken tortilla Soup

3:00 pm: Handful of nuts

7:00 pm: Chicken avocado mixed green salad

8:00 pm: Begin fasting

Day 17

8:00 am: Lemon water

8:30 am: Skip

12:00 pm: Chocolate peanut butter shake

3:00 pm: Roll fried zuchinni + smoke salmon

7:00 pm: Beef Stroganoff over Cauliflower mash

8:00 pm: Begin fasting

Day 18

8:00 am: Apple cider vinegar drink

8:30 am: Skip

12:00 pm: Tuna Avocado salad wrap

3:00 pm: Hummus + raw vegie sticks

7:00 pm: Asian fried "noodles"

8:00 pm: Begin fasting

Day 19

8:00 am: Lemon water

8:30 am: Skip

12:00 pm: Egg salad

3:00 pm: Piece of dark chocolate

7:00pm: Salmon kale salad

8:00 pm: Begin fasting

Day 20

8:00 am: Black coffee

8:30 am: Skip

12:00 pm: Turkey chili

3:00 pm: Organic Edamame

7:00 pm: Grilled chicken salad

8:00 pm: Begibn fasting

Day 21

8:00 am: Apple cider vinegar drink

12:00 pm: Grilled salmon salad

3:00 pm: Dark chocolate bark

7:00 pm: Chicken tortilla soup

8:00 pm: Begin fasting

CONCLUSION

Many women over 50 discover intermittent fasting is a smart approach to losing weight. Due to slow metabolism, losing weight at this age might be challenging. In addition, insulin resistance makes it more difficult for your body to digest sugars and carbohydrates.

For women over 50, intermittent fasting has various health advantages. You can benefit from improved heart health and diabetes control in addition to weight loss.

However, not everyone should practice intermittent fasting. If you decide to try it, be on the lookout for negative symptoms like headache, hunger pangs, or low energy. IF might not be the greatest weight reduction strategy for you if this is happening and does not get better within a week or two.

Before starting an intermittent fasting diet, talk to a nutritionist to lower the chance of adverse effects and figure out what's ideal for your goals.

Made in the USA
Coppell, TX
06 November 2022